HEALING
BREAKTHROUGHS

HEALING
BREAKTHROUGHS

Over 200 Up-to-the-Minute
Remedies and Cures
That Can Save Your Life

BY ISADORE ROSENFELD, M.D.
America's Most Trusted Doctor

RODALE

Notice

This book is intended as a reference volume only, not as a medical manual. The information given here is designed to help you make informed decisions about your health. It is not intended as a substitute for any treatment that may have been prescribed by your doctor. If you suspect that you have a medical problem, we urge you to seek competent medical help.

Mention of specific companies, organizations, or authorities in this book does not imply endorsement by the author or publisher, nor does mention of specific companies, organizations, or authorities imply that they endorse this book, its author, or the publisher.

Internet addresses and telephone numbers given in this book were accurate at the time it went to press.

Printed in the United States of America
Rodale Inc. makes every effort to use acid-free ∞, recycled paper ♻.

Cover and book design by Drew Frantzen

Library of Congress Cataloging-in-Publication Data

Rosenfeld, Isadore.
    Healing breakthroughs : over 200 up-to-the-minute remedies and cures that can save your life / by Isadore Rosenfeld.
        p.   cm.
    Includes index.
    ISBN 1–57954–969–1 hardcover
    1. Medicine, Popular.   I. Title.
    RC81.R8287   2004
    616—dc22   2004005676

2   4   6   8   10   9   7   5   3   1   hardcover

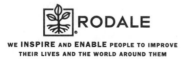
RODALE

WE **INSPIRE** AND **ENABLE** PEOPLE TO IMPROVE
THEIR LIVES AND THE WORLD AROUND THEM

FOR MORE OF OUR PRODUCTS
WWW.**RODALESTORE**.COM
(800) 848-4735

For my Camilla—again.

Wife, mother, granny, friend—and my continuing inspiration for almost half a century! (She was only a kid when it all began.)

CONTENTS

• • • • • • • • •

Parkinson's Disease

Pneumonia

Premenstrual Syndrome

Prostate Enlargement

Psoriasis

Rickets

Rosacea

Sexual Dysfunction

Sexually Transmitted Diseases

Shingles

Sinusitis

ACKNOWLEDGMENTS

· · · · · · · · ·

Special thanks to my superb editor, Leah Flickinger, for her vital role in the preparation of this book. Intelligent, relentlessly hard-working, perceptive, possessed of great judgment—and fun. I didn't really mind her incessant phone calls and e-mails designed, I know, to make sure we met all the deadlines. She deserves an honorary M.D.!

Special thanks also to my friend and agent Joni Evans who, with her usual perspicacity, has made this book possible. She worked with Leah and me on every stage of the book and her advice was, as usual, indispensable.

The value of a resource such as this book depends on meticulous confirmation of the facts presented. I am very grateful for the help provided me by my publisher, who assigned an extremely knowledgeable fact-checker to this project. Christina Bilheimer has, with great devotion and skill, ascertained the accuracy of the information on these pages.

Finally, I am both grateful and in awe of the genius and work of the many scientists, doctors, and researchers whose findings I have reported in these pages. Hope should spring eternal for the sick because of the dedication of these men and women to the welfare of mankind.

INTRODUCTION

. . . .

I remember when patients to whom I offered a choice of treatments would turn me down with, "You're the doctor. It's up to you. What do I know about medicine?" How times have changed! Most people now insist on having some input into what procedures they will agree to, whether or not to have an operation, and what side effects they will put up with from the medication that has been prescribed. Most physicians welcome such participation these days. Those who don't run the risk of having more leisure time as their practices dwindle.

After practicing medicine for more than 50 years, I am convinced that patients *should* be involved in their own medical care. For one thing, your body is continually sending important signals, not to your doctor but to *you*. Who better to interpret them than *you*, provided, of course, that you have learned something about what they can mean? (A little knowledge is not a dangerous thing as far as your health is concerned. In fact, the more, the better.) No matter what your medical problem happens to be, your input into how it should be evaluated and treated can make a big difference in its outcome.

There are other reasons for you to be informed and medically up-to-date. Progress is being made in all areas of medicine virtually every day. Theories once held sacred are being abandoned and replaced by totally new ones. Want some examples? Remember when post-menopausal women were urged to have hormone replacement therapy? Remember when no "reputable" doctor would have anything to do with the Atkins diet? Going back a little further, it's hard to believe that when I was in medical school, I was taught that high cholesterol is nothing to worry about and that high blood pressure is not dangerous. We used to keep heart attack patients on complete bed rest for 6 weeks, as a result of which many died of pulmonary embolism (blood clots to the lungs). All that has changed because medicine has evolved and continues to make incredible progress—in ideas, in techniques, and in treatment. You *and* your doctor should keep abreast of them.

I have written this book to make available to you the latest advances in many different fields of medicine—cardiology, oncology, gynecology, neurology, nutrition, pediatrics, psychiatry, and others—so that you can discuss with your physician what's relevant to you. If there has been an important breakthrough in the diagnosis or treatment of a disease, chances are you'll find it in these pages. Sometimes it's still being evaluated but seems promising, in which case you can follow its development with your doctor and know about it as soon as it's available.

Another reason to be informed and up-to-date has to do not so much with your health as with your health-insurance coverage. It's sad but true that your carrier has the last word on what tests and treatments will be approved. These decisions are based not on your welfare but on their cost. So it's critical that you know what tests and therapies are *best* for you and to insist on them—regardless of the expense to the third-party payer. That's your legal right!

Why, it may not even be too late for you to become a doctor yourself. Frankly, I have been trying all these years to turn my readers into an entirely new entity, "patient-doctors." Read this book carefully. You may be destined to become one.

ALCOHOLISM

. . . .

New Hope for Alcoholics

ACCORDING TO THE NATIONAL INSTITUTES OF HEALTH, 1 in every 13 American adults "abuses alcohol" or is an "alcoholic." (I have never understood the difference between these two definitions.) In my opinion, that figure is too low. I believe that more of us engage in binge drinking or drink heavily on a regular basis. I suspect that those who have an alcohol problem, or a potential one, may rationalize it to themselves and others, but in their heart of hearts they know that they need help. The tragedy is that they do not always ask for it and when they do, it's not always available or effective.

Here's a simple self-test to help you recognize a drinking problem. Ask yourself the following four questions:

• Have you ever felt you should cut down on your drinking?

• Do people annoy you when they criticize your drinking?

• Do you ever feel bad or guilty about your drinking?

• Do you need an eye-opener first thing in the morning to steady your nerves or get rid of a hangover?

If you answered yes to even one of these questions, you may have a drinking problem and you should look more closely into it, especially if other members of your immediate family have one too.

Although there is no cure for alcoholism, there are steps you can take to cope with it. For example, support groups such as Alcoholics Anonymous have helped many problem drinkers marital and psychological counseling also may be useful. When all else fails, check into a detoxification program. (Unfortunately, no matter what they do about it some 50 percent of alcoholics eventually go back to drinking after treatment.)

Many problem drinkers look to prescription medications for help with their problem. Three drugs are available:

1. **Antabuse (disulfiram)** makes you so sick that if you dare to drink while you're on it, you're terrified ever to booze again. It sounds good on paper, but Antabuse is not prescribed much anymore—for two reasons. Some of its adverse effects are severe and can harm the alcoholic, especially if he or she has some other underlying disease. More commonly, however, having tasted the wrath that can befall them if they drink while on Antabuse, most drinkers stay with the booze and avoid the medication. The cure is worse than the disease!

2. **Naltrexone**, originally introduced to control cravings for heroin and other narcotics, was approved by the FDA for keeping people off alcohol once they've quit. However, its ef-

fectiveness is disputed. One study found it to be of no use at all; another claimed success in one-third to one-half of cases. I've found its benefit to be limited among my patients.

3. **Acamprosate** is available in Europe but not yet in the United States. It acts on neurotransmitters in the brain to control the desire to drink. It helps in some cases.

HERE'S WHAT'S NEW

Researchers at the University of Texas Health Science Center in San Antonio have discovered that topiramate (marketed as Topamax), an approved antiseizure drug made from a naturally occurring sugar and used to treat epilepsy, appears to be much more effective in helping alcoholics quit drinking than any other drug available. According to their paper, published in the journal *The Lancet*, topiramate works by washing away excess dopamine, a chemical in the brain that enhances the craving for alcohol.

The researchers studied 103 heavy drinkers (men who regularly consumed more than five drinks a day and women who took more than four), all of whom had already tried and failed Alcoholics Anonymous, drug therapy, psychotherapy, and rehabilitation clinics. Fifty-five subjects were given oral topiramate; the remaining 48, a placebo. At the end of the study, 24 percent of those taking the topiramate had abstained completely for 1 month, compared with only 4 percent of the placebo group. Another plus for topiramate was that it improved abnormal liver function caused by alcohol excess in some patients. It also lifted mood and relieved anxiety symptoms.

Topiramate differs from all other antialcohol regimens, when judged by the duration of abstinence. Another plus is that patients on topiramate do not have to abstain completely and if they do continue to drink, they do so less than before. After all, 2 drinks are better and safer than 10. On all these accounts topiramate appears to be more effective than either naltrexone or acamprosate.

Although long-term use of topiramate by epileptics is generally safe, there are possible complications. This drug can worsen glaucoma; it can also interfere with the body's heat-regulating mechanism. Several cases of overheating and dehydration have been reported in kids being treated for epilepsy. Some questions have also been raised about topiramate's adverse effect on cognition (memory and thinking processes).

Although researchers will likely continue to evaluate this medication, experts are already hailing it as "a major scientific advance in the treatment of alcoholism." In fact, investigators are also assessing it for the treatment of obesity.

THE BOTTOM LINE

Topiramate appears to be more effective than other drugs currently available for treating alcohol addiction on the basis of results in one well-controlled study, and more will surely follow. It is already on the market (albeit for another purpose), so if you or a loved one has a severe alcohol problem and other therapies have failed, a doctor can prescribe topiramate for you.

ALZHEIMER'S DISEASE

• • • • • • • • •

The Latest News on Prevention

ABOUT FOUR MILLION AMERICANS are estimated to have Alzheimer's disease (AD). The symptoms of this degenerative brain disorder can be so subtle that many who are already in its early stages choose to deny them and so go undiagnosed and untreated. We used to deal with impotence in much the same way. "Impotent? Who, me? Naw. I'm just overworked." Then came Viagra, and suddenly millions of men who had deluded their partners, their doctors, and even themselves into believing they were sexual athletes began lining up for this new prescription. If and when there is a similar break-through for Alzheimer's, I predict that the current estimate of four million will escalate well into the double-digit millions. As it stands, the aging baby boomers are expected to raise that number to 14 million in the next few years.

5

Although its incidence is rising, AD is by no means a new disease. Ancient Greeks and Romans described it thousands of years ago. Alzheimer's is named after a German doctor, Alois Alzheimer, who in 1908 discovered twisted strands of fiber in the brains of some persons with "mental illness." These "neurofibrillary tangles" remain the only objective proof of Alzheimer's—and they're found only at autopsy.

Not until 75 years later did scientists discover that the characteristic Alzheimer's plaques contain beta amyloid, a string of 40 or more amino acids whose parent protein is called amyloid precursor protein (APP). This observation may turn out to be very important because researchers are now testing a vaccine that prevents this protein from forming. If it works, it may cure or prevent Alzheimer's. The tangles also contain another protein, called tau, which also is being studied.

Alzheimer's is not an immediate threat to life. Some patients survive for 20 years or more. However, many do die a few years after the diagnosis is made, usually from pneumonia or some other disease. AD costs Americans $100 billion a year, whether its victims are cared for at home or in nursing facilities.

AD is *not* an inevitable consequence of aging nor is it a vascular brain disease. Although it bears no relation to a stroke, repeated small strokes that damage the brain can cause senile dementia, whose symptoms resemble those of AD and are often mistaken for them. Yes, you are more likely to develop it as you grow older, but there is no such thing as "natural" senility. When you "lose" your mind at any age, it's because some disease or disorder has affected it. Alzheimer's is the most common of several such conditions.

The memory loss and other behavioral abnormalities of AD can usually be accurately assessed by neurological and psychiatric tests. Some of these are as simple as asking a patient, "What's the date, the day of the week, the year, and who's the President of the United States?" However, since no objective test currently exists to diagnose Alzheimer's *with certainty* while one is alive, everyone suspected of having it should undergo a careful neurological and medical evaluation to rule out the various other disorders that can produce similar symptoms.

High blood pressure, well documented as a cause of heart attack and stroke, is another risk factor for AD, especially in people over age 75. This strengthens the argument for treating elevated blood pressure as vigorously in the elderly as in the young.

HERE'S WHAT'S NEW

New observations about risk factors for Alzheimer's, how to predict it, and what to do to prevent it are frequently in the news. This past year, several large studies reached several important conclusions.

Researchers at Rush-Presbyterian/St. Luke's Medical Center in Chicago found that diets rich in saturated fat are associated with a greater risk for Alzheimer's. People who regularly consumed the most saturated fat were 2.3 times more likely to have Alzheimer's than those whose diets were lowest in saturated fats. (Meats and dairy products contain the most amount of saturated fats.)

By the same token, foods rich in monounsaturated and polyunsaturated fats reduce the risk. Examples of monounsaturated fats are olive and canola oils; the richest (and healthiest) sources of polyunsaturated fat (omega-3 fatty acids) are fatty fish, as well as plant and vegetable oils high in alpha-linoleic acid and linoleic acid (corn and safflower oils). A deficiency of these acids has been implicated in several mental disorders other than Alzheimer's.

An elevated homocysteine level is also a predictor of Alzheimer's disease. Thus far lowering or normalizing homocysteine has not been shown to make a difference. However, it remains an important marker of vascular disease. When elevated, all known factors should be vigorously attacked.

Certain genes are known to be associated with a higher incidence of AD. Still, you may have the gene and never develop AD, or you may not have it and get the disease anyway. However, there is one gene, the apolipoprotein E gene, that does appear to have significant predictive value for AD. Its presence is associated with an almost threefold incidence of the disease, but only in whites, not in African-Americans.

Recent studies suggest that the antioxidant vitamins C and E taken together protect against AD. A lifelong diet rich in folate (present in cereals, bread, and leafy green vegetables) appears to protect the brain in later years. For this and other reasons, I usually prescribe 400 micrograms of folic acid (the supplemental form of folate) to all my adult patients.

Research continues to emphasize the protective effect of two types of drugs: the statins that lower cholesterol and aspirin and other nonsteroidal anti-inflammatory drugs (NSAIDs) such as Motrin (ibuprofen) and Aleve (naproxen). However, these medications have no effect after symptoms of the disease have appeared.

Supplements of testosterone, the male hormone, have been shown to slow the formation of beta amyloid, present in the plaques of patients with Alzheimer's. Elderly men with AD who were given testosterone improved measurably. It's still too early to recommend this therapy to everyone, but it's worth discussing with your doctor. If the doctor balks, refer him or her to the research conducted by Dr. Gunnar Gouras at Weill Cornell Medical College in Ithaca, New York.

The latest research indicates that in postmenopausal women over age 65, estrogen-progesterone replacement therapy actually raises the risk of Alzheimer's disease and induces milder memory loss as well. Earlier studies had already implicated hormone replacement therapy as contributing to heart disease and stroke.

So, if you have a family history of Alzheimer's or have been tested for the gene and have been found to have it, I suggest a daily NSAID for prevention (even though many people with this gene never develop Alzheimer's—and vice versa).

THE BOTTOM LINE

I am not keen to learn whether I carry the genes that are likely to cause Alzheimer's sometime in the future. What's the point? There is nothing I can do about it at this point except follow the diet I describe above. I do that anyway. Learning that I have a good chance of losing my marbles when I get older simply would take the pleasure out of life while I still have them.

In addition to modifying your diet, the other steps to take for preventing AD are to keep your blood pressure normal and your cholesterol down. Statin drugs—the prototype of which is Lipitor (atorvastatin), though there are many others—not only lower high cholesterol but also appear to have a protective anti-inflammatory effect against AD. Also, the same anti-inflammatory properties of NSAIDs, are believed to delay or prevent AD, although they have no impact on symptoms once the disease has begun. So if you are caring for someone with Alzheimer's, NSAIDs will relieve chronic pain, but won't help senile dementia. Watch out for gastrointestinal bleeding, a common side effect of these drugs, especially in the elderly. Several studies, from such highly regarded institutions as the University of Washington in Seattle and Johns Hopkins University in Baltimore, have shown the effectiveness of NSAIDs in the *prevention* of Alzheimer's. Subjects who took any one of these agents daily for at least 2 years had a 73 percent reduced risk of developing Alzheimer's.

Aspirin was also beneficial but not to the same degree. Its daily use was found to reduce the subsequent risk of Alzheimer's by only 13 percent. Finally, testosterone replacement therapy may help older men who suffer from AD.

DHEA for Alzheimer's? Forget about It!

IF YOU LIKE TO BROWSE THE INTERNET, you likely are familiar with the "wonder hormone" called dehydroepiandrosterone (DHEA). There are literally hundreds of Web sites, in almost every language, devoted to promoting this miraculous product. And you won't have any problem getting as much of it as you want without a prescription.

DHEA is made by the adrenal glands that sit atop the kidneys. No one knows for sure what its function really is. The body makes little of it very early in life. Then, starting at about age 6, its production increases, peaking in the mid-twenties. (Men always have a little more than women.) From then on, it's all downhill. By age 75, both sexes have only 20 percent of the DHEA that they did 50 years earlier.

What an opportunity for "health" product entrepreneurs! Never mind trying to figure out why the body makes so much less DHEA as we age. That would take too long. Instead, these distributors simply assume because we have tons of DHEA when we're young and healthy, but by age 75 have very little, that taking lots and lots of it as we grow older will help us stay (or feel) young. Many thousands of people have fallen for this sales pitch, and DHEA is selling by the carload.

The FDA does not regulate DHEA, because they've designated it a "dietary supplement" not a drug. That can mean trouble for consumers. In a recent analysis of 16 DHEA products sold in the United States, one was found to contain absolutely none of the hormone, two had only a trace, and the DHEA content in the remaining 13 ranged from 69 to 150 percent of what the label claimed!

In experiments on mice and rats DHEA does appear to have a beneficial effect. However, there's a big difference between rodents and people. For starters, these animals produce only 1/10,000th the amount of DHEA that we do.

The results of studies on humans have been mixed—some have been favorable, others have not. Does that mean we should just take the hormone?

As I mentioned previously, we don't really understand DHEA's function. It may be simply a waste product of hormonal production. However, it eventually ends up as estrogen and testosterone. The FDA calls it the "mother hormone." (Saddam Hussein might have referred to it as "the mother of all hormones.") Taking extra DHEA means being saddled with more estrogen and testosterone, which may increase the risk of developing hormone-based cancers (of the breast in women and of the prostate in men). That's one important reason I do not recommend DHEA for *any* patient. And until the FDA begins supervising its production, you're buying a pig in the poke with every bottle you purchase.

HERE'S WHAT'S NEW

Acting on the observation that in some studies DHEA did improve memory in older mice, researchers at the University of California at San Francisco evaluated this effect in 58 people with Alzheimer's disease. This was a double-blind study in which half the participants received a placebo. Every patient was tested for thinking and memory function for 6 months. The results? An insignificant benefit in the DHEA-treated group after 3 months but, by 6 months, no major difference between the treated patients and those who received a placebo.

THE BOTTOM LINE

The results of this small study do not justify using DHEA to improve memory among the elderly. Until more research results are in, I wouldn't recommend this hormone for any reason. There are other, better ways to feel young—exercise and mental stimulation being among the most important.

WHAT THE DOCTOR ORDERED?

WHAT ABOUT GINKGO BILOBA? ● Ginkgo biloba is a best-selling feel-good herb. Complain about anything, and most complementary medicine enthusiasts will recommend ginkgo. It's a powerful antioxidant that has been used for centuries to treat a host of ailments. In the United States, it is especially popular for improving cognition (thinking and memory), and some doctors, especially those with a bent toward alternative medicine, recommend it for people with Alzheimer's disease (AD).

In my book *Dr. Rosenfeld's Guide to Alternative Medicine*, published in 1996, I too suggested ginkgo for this purpose because a study by the New York Institute for Medical Research found evidence of some cognitive improvement in AD patients taking it. Also, it appeared that ginkgo increases blood flow to the brain. Since then, the validity of the New York findings has been questioned, and proof of any major benefit from ginkgo remains sparse. However, there are several studies in progress to evaluate ginkgo and, who knows, they may show that it does help.

HERE'S WHAT'S NEW • Several healthy patients of mine who don't have even the slightest evidence of AD take ginkgo to improve their memory and "thinking processes." Recent studies suggest that it won't help a bit. Researchers at Williams College in Williamstown, Massachusetts, with a grant from the National Institutes of Health, conducted a well-designed, double-blind, randomized, controlled trial to determine whether ginkgo improved memory in 230 physically active and mentally healthy volunteers older than age 60. Half of the subjects took a 40-milligram tablet of ginkgo three times a day; the others were given a placebo. At the end of 6 weeks, all were tested for verbal and nonverbal learning, memory, attention, concentration, and expressive language (finding the right word). There was no difference whatsoever between the two groups.

Claims that herbal supplements offer miracle benefits are often not backed up by scientific testing. Even when they are, you still don't know what you're getting when you pick a bottle off a shelf, because it may not contain what the label says it does.

ConsumerLab, an independent testing laboratory in White Plains, New York, analyzes various products for a fee. In recent tests on various brands of ginkgo, they found that only 22 percent met quality standards. Most contained only one-fifth of the active ingredient claimed on the label. This is a marked drop from the 75 percent that had passing grades in 1999. Only two of the nine brands randomly selected passed the test—Maxi Ginkgo Biloba and Nature's Way Ginkgold. A third company, which requested and paid for its product—Nutrilite Ginkgo Biloba—to be analyzed also met the standard.

Here's the quandary: As the ginkgo debate continues among scientists, consumers face the additional possibility that, even if the herb does work, they have no way of knowing whether the brand they use contains enough of the active ingredient.

THE BOTTOM LINE • If you're healthy, don't waste your money on ginkgo. This herb probably won't do anything for you, even though it may increase blood flow to various organs of the body, including the brain. However because there are so few treatment alternatives for Alzheimer's, I see no harm in someone with AD taking ginkgo even though to date it has not proven to have an effect on the disease. Remember, however, that this herb is a mild blood thinner, so use it with caution if you're also taking an anticoagulant; discontinue both before having any surgery. •

ARTHRITIS

· · · · · · · · ·

Does Tylenol Really Help Osteoarthritis?

OSTEOARTHRITIS, the degeneration of the body's joints due to wear and tear over the years, is a major cause of disability and pain in older men and women. Most patients require painkillers ranging from something as simple as aspirin and Tylenol (acetaminophen) to non-steroidal anti-inflammatory drugs (NSAIDs) to potent narcotics. Always start with the least potent drugs.

Tylenol is generally safe and non–habit-forming, which is why it is available over the counter and usually recommended as the first drug to try for relief of "the aches and pains of minor arthritis," as referred to in the TV commercials. Although the drug is easier on the stomach than many NSAIDs and aspirin, Tylenol overdose is one of the leading causes of poisoning cases that end up in emergency rooms in this country. Exceeding the recommended dose can hurt the liver, especially if you have a drinking problem or any kind of liver disease.

Questions have recently been raised about Tylenol's effectiveness despite its widespread use, since osteoarthritic pain is now believed to be caused not only by long-term joint use but also by inflammation. Unlike the NSAIDs and the newer COX-2 inhibitors, such as Celebrex (celecoxib), Vioxx (rofecoxib), and Bextra (valdecoxib), Tylenol does not reduce inflammation. It acts on the nerves that transmit pain.

The manufacturer insists that Tylenol is effective, and so do millions of patients. Are they right, or is the benefit they describe all in the head?

HERE'S WHAT'S NEW

Researchers at the Rush-Presbyterian/St. Luke's Medical Center in Chicago compared the efficacy of Tylenol and anti-inflammatory drugs in 82 men and women with painful osteoarthritis of the knee. One-third of the subjects were given 1,000 milligrams of generic acetaminophen four times a day, another third received 75 milligrams of the NSAID Voltaren (diclofenac) twice daily. The rest took a placebo. Neither the researchers nor the patients knew what they were getting.

Using standard measures to determine pain and the stage of the arthritis at the beginning of the study and again after 2 and 12 weeks, researchers assessed the results of each treatment. Guess what? Those taking the NSAID significantly improved, whereas patients on either acetaminophen or placebo did not. What's more, there was *no* difference in the results obtained between the placebo and acetaminophen groups! I can understand a better result from the NSAID than from the Tylenol, but no benefit whatsoever from the Tylenol really surprises me. The researchers concluded that "acetaminophen use in subjects with osteoarthritis of the knee should be reconsidered pending further studies."

THE BOTTOM LINE

I don't expect this to be the last word on the subject. Tylenol is so popular and so widely used that other studies will certainly test how well it relieves osteoarthritis pain. For now, if Tylenol works for you, I recommend you stay with it. If, however, your pain is not responding, don't assume that it's because your arthritis is bad or getting worse. Don't increase the dose of Tylenol and run the risk of toxicity. Switch to an NSAID and take it, as directed, *after* meals or with milk, to avoid stomach irritation.

A final piece of advice: Don't confuse the painkilling properties of Tylenol with its ability to reduce an elevated temperature. The osteoarthritis study did not address the latter problem. If you're running a fever, Tylenol will lower it.

WHAT THE DOCTOR ORDERED?

ARNICA FOR PAIN ● When I was an undergraduate student at McGill University in Montreal, I was passionate about football (watching not playing). My admiration and envy for friends on the team changed to sympathy in the locker room after the game when I saw how bruised and battered they were. Yet, their spirits seemed undiminished as they applied arnica compresses to their aching bodies. (Some also took it in homeopathic tablet form.)

Years later, while in medical school, I was surprised that I was taught nothing about this miracle medication, also called leopard's bane. After graduation and throughout my residency, I never once saw it used in the hospital, where pain of all kinds is treated. Was there some conspiracy by those in evidence-based medicine against all the "wisdom" offered by many "natural" therapies used throughout the ages? Those stubborn teachers of mine, and later my colleagues in practice, kept insisting on proof of effectiveness before prescribing or recommending any medication, including arnica, whether or not it required a prescription.

In later years, as my immediate relationship to the football field and my contact with its players waned, I forgot about arnica. I treated my pain patients with the gamut of conventional agents ranging from aspirin and Tylenol (acetaminophen) all the way to OxyContin (oxycodone), depending on how much they hurt.

Then, a few years ago, I wrote a book called *Dr. Rosenfeld's Guide to Alternative Medicine.* I based it on a careful review of the scientific literature about, among many other things, arnica. The remedy is still widely used, especially by athletes, just as it was when I was in college some 50 years ago. But in all my research on the subject I could find no convincing evidence that it really works. In 1998, findings from eight well-controlled trials reported in the *Archives of Surgery* concluded that arnica exerts only a placebo effect despite innumerable testimonials to its effectiveness.

I was at my local health food store the other day to buy some glucosamine and chondroitin for my aching knees when I saw some arnica on a shelf. I asked the owner how well it was selling. "Great," he replied, "as always." I asked him whether his customers preferred the tablets or the topical solutions. "Both," he answered, "but I think the tablets are better."

I decided to review the subject again, this time on the Internet, because I had exhausted all my scientific sources when I wrote my book on alternative medicine. I was amazed to find at site after site, almost all of which were hosted by purveyors of the product or homeopathic practitioners, claims that arnica cures or improves the following conditions, to list just a few: coronary artery disease, a weak immune system, bumped and bruised tissue, arthritis pain, chapped lips, acne, irritated nostrils, fever, dry skin, fluid retention, dry cough (it's apparently an expectorant, too), arteries in spasm, and fatigue (it's also a stimulant). Wow! What a track record for just a single herb! No wonder homeopaths are so keen about it.

I was curious to see what our stick-in-the-mud FDA had to say about arnica. It seems that the government strongly believes that oral preparations of arnica, other than the diluted homeopathic strengths, are unsafe and contain substances that can actually hurt the heart and vascular system, cause violent toxic gastroenteritis, nervous disturbances, intense muscle weakness, contact dermatitis, collapse, and death. So why aren't these toxic oral preparations banned? Because they aren't classified as drugs. Considered "natural supplements," they are not under FDA control. Although the FDA does not question the safety of the topical applications of arnica or the homeopathic oral preparations, it does not endorse their effectiveness either.

HERE'S WHAT'S NEW • The following is for all the arnica enthusiasts who swear by both its oral and topically applied forms. Researchers at the University of Exeter and the Royal Devon and Exeter Hospital in the United Kingdom conducted a rigorous double-blind study of three groups of patients with carpal tunnel syndrome (a painful disorder of the wrist) who took arnica by mouth for 1 week before and 2 weeks after surgery. One group was given high-potency arnica tablets; another, low-potency tablets; the remaining third, a placebo. Neither the participants nor the doctors treating them knew who was getting what. The patients filled out standard pain-assessment questionnaires throughout the experiment. Their wrists were also photographed at every stage to document the degree of swelling and exact shades of bruising.

After all evidence was in, the researchers concluded that there was "no significant difference" among the 3 groups in terms of bruising, swelling, pain, and the number of painkillers used. There were no toxic effects either.

The researchers recommend that if you hurt for whatever reason, you should use more effective treatment and save money by not buying homeopathic arnica. When asked to explain the large number of anecdotal kudos for this herb, they point out that no two people react to pain in the same way. Those who normally recover quickly anyway and take arnica rave about it to their friends. The nonresponders simply keep mum—and that's how a legend is born and perpetuated.

In all fairness, most homeopaths do not recommend the herb for postoperative pain, so this study should not be taken as a definitive assessment of arnica's use in mild to moderate muscle strain or bruising.

In this study, published in the *Journal of the Royal Society of Medicine*, only oral arnica was used. I'm sorry that they did not evaluate topical arnica. I just can't believe that the entire McGill football team was wrong.

THE BOTTOM LINE • If friends on your college or home football team are applying arnica to their bruised bodies and are happy with it, they should stay with it. It can do no harm unless they develop contact dermatitis, and they'll know that soon enough. However, neither you nor they should take arnica by mouth (other than the diluted homeopathic preparations labeled as such) because, as far as the FDA is concerned, it is dangerous. •

ASTHMA

· · · · · · · · ·

Respect the Common Cold

VIRUSES THAT CAUSE THE COMMON COLD (of which there are more than 200) must have an inferiority complex. Even though they make millions of adults and kids miserable at least once a year, no one really worries about them. The flu, a migraine, diarrhea—usually warrant a day off, but you're expected to carry on when you have only a "cold." Try telling your boss that you're staying home because that's what you have! Even worse, try saying that you aren't coming to work because your *child* has a cold!

According to a recent study, cough medications and decongestants were found to be of no use whatsoever in treating the common cold (see page 76). And don't bother asking your doctor for an antibiotic (which, incidentally, most people do and sometimes even succeed in getting). You're sure to receive a lecture about how antibiotics don't work against viruses and why it's important to save them for when you're "really sick."

HERE'S WHAT'S NEW

It turns out that the common cold can pack a more powerful punch than we thought—at least for children with asthma. Researchers at the University of Iowa College of Medicine are strongly advising parents of asthmatic children to keep oral steroids handy and to give them to their kids at the first sign of a cold. The scientists have found that doing so greatly reduces the risk of an asthma emergency down the line. Any kind of respiratory infection—from "just a cold" to the "real" flu—can trigger serious asthma attacks. Kids younger than age 5 are five times more likely to be hospitalized with the complications of asthma unless they are promptly treated with an oral steroid (the drugs most commonly used for this purpose are prednisone or prednisolone)—and the sooner, the better. That means always keeping some on hand. Such prompt treatment can prevent up to 90 percent of emergency asthma visits to the hospital.

Results from a related short-term study also reassure parents not to worry about the complications of oral steroids used briefly from time to time for the treatment of acute respiratory symptoms. Researchers at McGill University Health Centre in Montreal found that these medications do not affect bone density or result in any difference in the growth or weight of children who received as many as 11 short courses of such therapy for as long as 1 year.

THE BOTTOM LINE

If you have an asthmatic child, keep a supply of oral steroids on hand. At the earliest signs of a cold, start treatment for a few days. The sooner you do so, the less likely your child will be to develop a severe asthma attack. Unless you have this medication readily available, symptoms that start after the pharmacies close on Saturday night may go untreated until Monday morning, when the drug stores reopen—and that's too long. Note, however, that this recommendation applies only to children with asthma—not all children.

When Asthma Doesn't Respond to Medication

SOME ASTHMATIC KIDS are in and out of emergency rooms with acute respiratory distress because their asthma hasn't responded to maximal doses of any medication. This resistance to conventional treatment has always been interpreted as evidence that their disease is severe.

We have long known that in many adult asthmatics, acid reflux from the stomach into the esophagus (gastroesophageal reflux disease or GERD) causes chronic cough and hoarseness independent of their respiratory disease. Indeed their asthma usually improves after the acid reflux is treated.

HERE'S WHAT'S NEW

Doctors at the West Jefferson Medical Center in New Orleans theorized that children with persistent moderate asthma who also have GERD might have fewer respiratory symptoms if their acid reflux were treated. They studied 46 asthmatic children, 27 of whom had GERD. They treated most of the latter group with either anti-GERD therapy, such as acid-suppressing drugs (proton pump inhibitors) or surgical correction for the few who needed it.

Here's how this therapy affected their asthma after 12 months: Overall, they needed 50 percent fewer bronchodilators. During the last 6 months of the study, 89 percent took no inhaled steroids whatsoever. None required leukotriene receptor antagonists (see page 26).

By contrast, asthmatic children whose GERD was not treated required the same respiratory medications they had taken all along. Even more interesting, eight of the children who did not have GERD but who chose to receive treatment for it anyway also required less anti-asthma medication.

THE BOTTOM LINE

No one really knows why treating GERD reduces symptoms of asthma. But the results of this study, published in *Chest* (the official peer-reviewed journal of the American College of Chest Physicians), strongly suggest that asthmatics who have GERD—and maybe even those who don't—should take medication that decreases the amount of acid produced by the stomach. Doing so appears to reduce the severity of their disease and the amount of anti-asthma medication required.

WHAT THE DOCTOR ORDERED?

THE HYGIENE HYPOTHESIS • For the past several years, doctors have wondered why the incidence of asthma and allergies has been rising, especially in developed countries such as the United States. One possible explanation is that, in keeping with our "higher standard of living," we compulsively overprotect our children against relatively harmless infectious organisms and irritants. Keeping bedrooms free from dust, mites, and molds, and scrupulously avoiding contact with other children who have colds and other infections may be the wrong thing to do.

HERE'S WHAT'S NEW • Asthma and allergy researchers at the National Jewish Medical and Research Center in Denver as well as specialists elsewhere believe that our emphasis on cleanliness and hygiene early in life is making us more vulnerable to asthma and allergies later on. In their opinion, children need some exposure to infectious organisms so that their immune systems can be prepared against more serious attacks when we're older. Overprotecting them early on leaves them with no experience in coping with relatively harmless irritants and infectious agents that normally stimulate antibody formation. This lack of protection may result in asthma and allergy years down the line.

The Denver research team found strong evidence to support the hygiene hypothesis with experiments on mice, a group of whom they injected with a bacterium that commonly causes pneumonia. Others received a placebo. Two weeks later, both groups were rendered allergic to an egg protein and their respective responses were evaluated. The animals that had been infected with the bacterium had a much milder reaction to the egg protein than did the controls. Their levels of gamma interferon (a synthetic version of a substance that the body produces naturally to help fight infections and tumors) were also higher than in the healthy, nonallergic animals.

Even though mice are not men, these doctors believe that this controlled experiment supports the hypothesis that sparing children a little dust and dirt—or even exposure to a bug or two—can leave them more allergic and vulnerable to more serious problems later on.

I discussed this theory with two of my grandchildren, ages 7 and 11, who had just been told to clean up their rooms. They heartily agree with the researchers and now beg to let a little dust accumulate here and there, especially in their own living quarters.

THE BOTTOM LINE • Once a person becomes asthmatic or allergic, it's important to avoid exposure to dust, mites, mold, and infection. However, early in life, small doses of these "contaminants" help the body's immune system develop antibodies when it's challenged later on. Keep your house clean, by all means, but don't overprotect your children. •

Newer Treatment Not Always Better

FOR YEARS, many people with mild to moderate asthma used inhaled corticosteroids, such as Flonase or Flovent (fluticasone propionate), to reduce the swelling and inflammation of the nasal and respiratory passages.

More recently, newer drugs called leukotriene receptor antagonists (like Singulair) have gained popularity in the United States and are commonly taken in place of inhaled steroids. Leukotrienes, like histamines, are substances released when the body is challenged by something to which it is allergic, and that cause the symptoms of allergy. Leukotriene receptor antagonists (LTRAs) are used in the same way as antihistamines to treat these symptoms.

The popularity of LTRAs may be the result of a combination of effective advertising and concern about the safety of inhaled steroids, often confused with the oral preparations. Large doses of the latter can cause serious adverse reactions when taken for prolonged periods of time; inhaled steroids do not.

Complementary (alternative) medicine devotees believe that homeopathic remedies also improve quality of life for people with mild to moderate asthma, even though most conventional health providers are not convinced of the benefits. Indeed, homeopathic remedies are given to 15 percent of asthmatic children in the United Kingdom. The number in this country is probably less but still substantial.

HERE'S WHAT'S NEW

Researchers at McGill University Health Centre found the newer nonsteroidal, antileukotrienes less effective than inhaled steroids. Adults with asthma so treated were 60 percent more likely to have flare-ups, awaken at night, and experience daytime symptoms.

Recently, the University of Exeter's department of complementary medicine conducted a double-blind study of 93 asthmatic children in southwest England. Homeopathic remedies prescribed by experienced, classically trained homeopaths and continued for 1 year were found to be no more effective than placebos.

THE BOTTOM LINE

If you have mild to moderate asthma that is well-controlled by an *inhaled* corticosteroid that you tolerate well, stay with it. Inhaled steroids are safer than the oral form. If you do decide to try an antileukotriene such as Singulair and it works, fine. If it doesn't, however, don't hesitate to go back to the inhaled steroids. They are safe, and their adverse effects are minimal.

If you've been thinking about homeopathy to help your asthma, it will leave you breathless. There are better ways to spend your time and money.

ATTENTION-DEFICIT HYPERACTIVITY DISORDER

· · · · · · · · ·

New Treatment, New Approach

ATTENTION-DEFICIT HYPERACTIVITY DISORDER (ADHD) is a common behavioral abnormality that starts in childhood, affects 4 to 6 percent of all Americans, and continues throughout life in up to two-thirds of all cases. Kids with ADHD can't focus their attention on anything for long, they're impulsive (if they want something, they must have it right away), and they can't sit still.

Is ADHD a disorder or simply a variant of normal behavior? Federal legislation has designated ADHD a disability, meaning that anyone so diagnosed is entitled to help—at school and at work. Digital imaging studies and positron emission tomography (PET) scans of the brains of people with ADHD have shown that areas that control attention and inhibit impulses are less active and use less sugar for energy than do other parts of the brain. Also, ADHD runs in families: If one family member has ADHD, there is a 25 to 35 percent chance that another will too, compared with only a 4 to 6 percent probability for someone in the general population.

Still, some doctors think that ADHD is overdiagnosed; others even deny that it's a disease. (We used to think that sugar was responsible for hyperactivity, but that's apparently true in only 5 percent of kids). There is also considerable (and occasionally passionate) disagreement about how to treat ADHD. Most observers agree that children with the classic signs of this disorder—fidgeting, squirming, talking a blue streak, blurting out answers to questions that haven't been asked—should have behavioral and cognitive therapy. However, many specialists have serious doubts about the overuse of stimulant medications, such as Ritalin (methylphenidate), Dexedrine (dextroamphetamine), and Adderall (dextroamphetamine/amphetamine). Some experts believe that Ritalin is responsible for addiction, that it disrupts growth hormone, and that it may cause physical damage to the brain. For these reasons, the following news is welcome.

HERE'S WHAT'S NEW

The FDA has approved a new drug, Strattera (atomoxetine), as a safe, effective treatment for ADHD for patients of any age. It is the first *nonstimulant* medication designated for this purpose. Strattera works by blocking the brain's reabsorption of norepinephrine, a neurotransmitter that sends messages between brain cells and regulates attention, impulsivity, and activity levels. The standard dose is one or two capsules a day, and adverse effects are minimal, typically involving some loss of appetite and, occasionally, an allergic reaction.

Another interesting study has concluded that children with ADHD respond better to medication if they also receive biofeedback therapy. These children had better attention spans and behavior ratings, as well as measurable improvement of images of their brain activity, than those who weren't. In some children, this improvement continued for 2 years after completing 40 sessions of biofeedback. The researchers conclude that biofeedback is especially helpful for kids who don't tolerate drugs well or who may have trouble stopping their medication because of a family history of addiction.

THE BOTTOM LINE

If your child (or you, for that matter) has been diagnosed with ADHD, is being treated with a stimulant drug, and is not happy with this therapy for whatever reason, you now have an alternative. Ask your doctor about nonstimulant Strattera. Also, consider a course of biofeedback therapy because it appears to enhance the effectiveness of medication.

BAD BREATH

• • • • • • • • • •

New Strategies for Fresher Breath

BREATH ALWAYS HAS SOME ODOR TO IT—sometimes even a pleasant one. Unfortunately, it also can be offensive. Bad breath (or halitosis) can result from many different causes. Following are the ones to think about first:

- Sinus infections, especially if accompanied by a postnasal drip

- Infected tonsils

- Chronic lung disease with mucus in the airways

- Kidney and liver disease (odorous waste products accumulate in the blood and circulate through the body causing bad breath to ensue when they are exhaled by the lungs)

- Infections in the mouth (teeth, gums, and tongue)

• Regular consumption of acidic foods, caffeine, and fish (garlic and onions cause only temporary halitosis)

Treating halitosis is big business. Pharmacies and health food stores offer a slew of products—special chewing gums, mints, mouthwashes, and sprays—all of which promise to "freshen" your breath (and allow you to use words that start with the letter *H* in intimate conversations). Few of them work for more than a couple of minutes. In fact, a mouthwash that contains alcohol may make things worse. Brushing your teeth more frequently won't help much either. The only effective way to control bad breath is to eliminate whatever is causing it.

HERE'S WHAT'S NEW

Researchers at Baskent University in Turkey have observed that patients with *H. pylori* infection of the stomach frequently have halitosis. (This bacterium commonly inhabits in the stomach and has been implicated as a possible cause of gastric ulcers, bleeding, and even cancer.) They studied 148 men and women with *H. pylori* and who had various gastrointestinal signs and symptoms, such as indigestion, bloating, and burping. About 60 percent of them also had halitosis. After their *H. pylori* was eradicated with the appropriate antibiotic, many of those with halitosis reported that their bad breath had cleared up. So, if your breath is offensive and you have stomach "trouble," ask your doctor to check you for *H. pylori* with a simple blood test or breath analysis. If the results are abnormal and there is no other explanation for the halitosis, have the *H. pylori* treated with an antibiotic. That may not only clean your breath but also help prevent more serious stomach problems later on.

Here's another way to freshen your breath. Researchers at Pace University in New York City and at the University of Illinois have found that a cup of tea can do the trick by fighting oral infection. In the Pace University study, when green tea was added to cultures of the bacteria that cause strep throat and tooth decay, it destroyed almost 100 percent of the organisms. The researchers believe that the polyphenol in tea acts on the bacteria. They suggest that toothpaste manufacturers add these polyphenols to toothpaste and mouthwash to protect the mouth against infection (and the bad breath that accompanies it).

In the University of Illinois study, researchers found that black tea reduced by 30 percent the growth of three types of mouth bacteria that cause bad breath. They suggest rinsing your mouth regularly with black tea to reduce plaque formation and halitosis caused by these bacteria.

THE BOTTOM LINE

If your bad breath persists even after you've eliminated some of its more common causes, have yourself checked for *H. pylori* (especially if you have chronic indigestion or other stomach complaints). Treatment of *H. pylori* requires 10 to 14 days of an antibiotic, several different regimens of which are available.

Being treated for *H. pylori* is the first course of action. Then, get into the habit of drinking tea—green or black. Both types contain polyphenols, which inhibit the growth of bacteria and viruses responsible for oral infection and bad breath. If you'd rather not drink the tea, just rinse your mouth regularly with it. It's a good mouthwash.

BODY ODOR

* * * * * * * * *

Yet Another Use for Botox—
Who Would Have Thought?

MANY YEARS AGO WHEN I WAS A MEDICAL STUDENT, we learned about a condition called botulism. Caused by a toxin from the bacterium *Clostridium botulinum*, this illness can lead to paralysis and even death. You get it by eating contaminated canned foods that have a low acid content, such as asparagus, green beans, beets, and corn (usually canned at home). The clostridium spores can also be present in honey.

There are only about 100 cases of botulism a year in the United States, so it's no surprise that I've never seen a case in all the years I've been practicing medicine. Still, I always think of botulism whenever I see a patient with any of its classic signs or symptoms—double vision, blurred vision, drooping eyelids, slurred speech, difficulty swallowing, severe dry mouth, and muscle weakness.

So imagine my shock a few years ago when I began hearing about all the wonderful things that this deadly poison can do. It has found respectability—even admiration and gratitude—under the commercial name Botox, a very, very diluted strength of which can help erase wrinkles when injected into the skin. Men and women are flocking to their cosmetic gurus for these facial Botox treatments. You can recognize someone who's had the procedure, by the bland, expressionless look not unlike the loss of facial expression in someone with Parkinson's disease. I'm not knocking Botox, mind you, because beauty is in the eyes of the beholder.

Botox has a more tangible upside than cosmetic results. It can help relieve migraine headaches by relaxing facial muscles (see page 249) and also can reduce excessive underarm perspiration when injected there.

HERE'S WHAT'S NEW

Chalk up another victory to this dreaded toxin. German researchers have discovered that Botox not only reduces underarm perspiration but also virtually eliminates its offensive odors. It isn't clear how it works; it may interfere with skin bacteria or act on the nerves of the sweat glands. Whatever the mechanism, it gets rid of the smell, and that's what counts.

THE BOTTOM LINE

If you're considering a facelift, ask about Botox first. If you have offensive underarm odors (bad enough so that your best friend tells you about it), try a variety of powerful antiperspirants first. But if none work and your social life is going down the drain, ask your doctor about Botox treatments.

But remember this: Whether for "beauty" or for treatment of any of the other disorders I've mentioned, this is not a one-shot deal—you need to receive Botox injections every few months for continued results. And it doesn't come cheap!

BREAST CANCER

· · · · · · · · ·

Minimize Your Risk with Ibuprofen

BREAST CANCER IS THE MOST COMMON MALIGNANCY in women in the United States (excluding nonmelanoma skin cancer) and the second leading cause of cancer deaths among them. In 2004, at least 200,000 new cases of invasive breast cancer will be diagnosed in this country and some 40,000 women will die. (Breast cancer will also strike close to 1,300 men this year, of whom 400 will die.)

Although early detection of breast cancer is the key to its successful treatment, preventing it is even more desirable. There are several risk factors that increase your chances of developing it. Here are the most important ones:

Age. The incidence of breast cancer increases with age. A female born today has one chance in 252 of developing breast cancer between ages 30 and 40; the risk is 1 in 68 between ages 40 and 50, and 1 in 27 between ages 60 and 70. By age 85, her lifetime chance of developing breast cancer is 1 in 8.

Genetics. About 10 percent of breast cancers are hereditary. If your mother, sister, or daughter had breast cancer, you're at twice the risk of developing it too. You can determine your genetic vulnerability by being tested for mutations of the BRCA1 and BRCA2 genes. Mutations of either gene indicate an increased risk of breast as well as ovarian cancers.

Previous breast cancer. A previous history of cancer in one breast triples or quadruples your chances of developing a recurrent cancer in the same breast or the other.

Hormones. The lifetime level of female hormone estrogen produced by the ovaries is believed to be directly related to the risk of breast cancer. Women who've had one or both ovaries removed are less likely to develop this cancer later on in life, and the longer your ovaries have been making estrogen, the greater your risk. Estrogen production drops during pregnancy. So if your estrogen supply has remained high because you've never had children, you're at higher risk for breast cancer. (That's presumably why nuns are so vulnerable to this malignancy.) Conversely, the more kids you've had and the earlier in life you had them, the lower your risk.

By the same token, 5 or more years of hormone replacement therapy raises the incidence of breast cancer. Whether taking birth control pills also does so is still under debate.

Drugs like Nolvadex (tamoxifen) suppress estrogen production or action and thus reduce the likelihood of breast cancer. Remember, however, that this drug increases the risk of uterine cancer, stroke, and blood clots in the veins, so consider the risk-benefit ratio before deciding whether to take it.

Radiation history. Radiation therapy also can predispose a person to cancer anywhere in the body, including the breast. If you received such radiation during childhood for any reason (Hodgkin's disease, thyroid problems, even acne), you may be more vulnerable to breast cancer. It's also a good reason to think twice about having children undergo routine dental or chest x-rays.

Unfortunately, you can't do much about such risk factors as your age or family history. But you do have control over some others. For example, reconsider hormone replacement therapy. Fewer women take it these days, not only because it raises the risk of cancer but also because earlier assessments of its benefits have not been substantiated (see page 243). As far as the Pill is concerned, the possibility of increased danger of breast cancer arising from its use is so small that it should not affect your decision to take it.

Various lifestyle modifications also can reduce your risk. Exercising regularly may lower your hormone levels; breastfeeding is also helpful. Drinking alcohol raises the risk somewhat. Cigarette smoking is bad for you for other reasons, and a study published in April 2001 found that smoking significantly increases the risk of breast cancer in women with a strong family history of breast and ovarian cancers.

Your diet is important on two accounts. First, gaining weight increases your risk, especially after menopause. Second, populations that eat a high-fat diet have a higher incidence of breast cancer.

If you have a host of significant risk factors such as a strong family history of breast cancer, ovarian cancer, or both as well as the presence of mutated BRCA1 and BRCA2 genes, you should consider having both breasts removed. Doing so reduces the risk of breast cancer by 90 percent. And don't worry about the cosmetic effect— you'd be surprised at how effectively sophisticated breast reconstruction techniques restore the appearance of the chest.

HERE'S WHAT'S NEW

An Ohio State University study of 80,000 postmenopausal women ages 50 to 79 revealed that those who took a single 200-milligram tablet of ibuprofen (the most popular brand names are Motrin and Advil) two or more times a week for at least 10 years reduced their risk of breast cancer by 49 percent. Aspirin worked too, but not quite as well. A single 325-milligram tablet reduced the incidence of breast cancer by 22 percent. This was true even for women with strong family histories and other risk factors. Tylenol (acetaminophen), a painkiller but not an anti-inflammatory, had no effect on the incidence of breast cancer.

The lead researcher on this study believes that anti-inflammatory drugs probably work against other cancers as well. In fact, other investigations have shown that anti-inflammatories help prevent cancers of the colon by 20 to 30 percent (and may also protect against heart attacks and Alzheimer's disease).

It's not entirely clear why anti-inflammatories have this protective effect. It may be that they prevent cancer by blocking harmful gene mutations and the spread of cancer cells, and may also speed the death of malignant cells.

THE BOTTOM LINE

The over-the-counter anti-inflammatory drug ibuprofen, taken only twice a week over a 10-year period, can reduce the incidence of this malignancy by almost half, as can a single aspirin tablet, albeit somewhat less effectively. Unless you have a bleeding disorder, gastrointestinal problems, allergic reaction to these drugs, or are taking anticoagulants, ask your doctor about the pros and cons of taking an NSAID—especially if you are at high risk for breast cancer.

Pregnancy Loss Not a Risk Factor

FOR MANY YEARS a National Cancer Institute (NCI) fact sheet stated that there is "no causal association between abortion and breast cancer." Then, toward the end of 2002, it revised that conclusion to read that any linkage between induced abortions and breast cancer was still "inconclusive."

Why was the possibility of a link between pregnancy loss and breast cancer raised in the first place? It was all highly theoretical. Here's the logic: There is an association between the duration of exposure to estrogen and the incidence of breast cancer. As mentioned earlier, the longer a woman has high concentrations of this hormone circulating in her body, the greater her risk of breast cancer. During pregnancy, those hormone levels fall—and that's good as far as breast cancer is concerned. Conversely, terminating a pregnancy for any reason raises the estrogen level. So, at least theoretically, an interrupted pregnancy could increase the risk of breast cancer later in life.

HERE'S WHAT'S NEW

Now, in an even newer version of the fact sheet, the NCI states that abortion, induced or spontaneous (the latter including miscarriage), is *not* associated with an increase in breast cancer risk.

Four substantial studies and a review of several earlier ones were evaluated at an NCI workshop in early 2003 by a specially appointed scientific panel. One study involving 1.5 million Danish women concluded that those who'd had induced abortions were not at increased risk of breast cancer. Earlier reports that suggested otherwise were determined to be flawed.

Absolving abortion of this stigma does not weaken the link between estrogen and breast cancer. This same panel also concluded that the more babies a woman has, and the younger she is when her first full-term baby is born, the less likely she is to develop breast cancer. Women who have never given birth have about the same risk of breast cancer as those who delivered their firstborns at age 30.

THE BOTTOM LINE

The number of terminated pregnancies a woman has had—whether induced or natural—has no bearing whatsoever on her risk of developing breast cancer later on. This fear should not prey on your mind. Regardless of your obstetrical history, every woman should be screened for breast cancer starting at age 40. How often to do so (and whether to be screened *before* age 40) depends on the presence of other risk factors.

WHAT THE DOCTOR ORDERED?

THE MAMMOGRAM DEBATE For years, routine mammography has been a "given" for most American women. That's because (1) breast cancer is a leading cause of death among them, (2) mammography detects many small cancers up to 2 years earlier than do manual breast examinations, and (3) early diagnosis increases the chance of a cure. So it would seem indisputable that vulnerable females, and all those age 40 and older, should have an annual mammogram. Right? Not necessarily, according to some observers.

Who dares challenge this advice? Lots of people. First, there are the "cost effectiveness" types, forever trying to determine how many lives mammography must save in order to make its routine use "worthwhile." Then there are the statisticians, analyzing numbers to determine how "reliable" the mammogram is in diagnosing breast cancer and whether screening really makes any difference to overall survival. There are also "experts" who question whether the mammogram is, in fact, the best way to diagnose breast cancer— and whether women shouldn't use another technique either instead of or in addition to it. Finally, some oncologists claim that early detection makes no difference in the long run for many breast cancers, and that there is plenty of time to treat tumors after they are large enough to be felt.

Each reservation about mammography has some validity. However, are they sufficiently relevant to preclude having an annual mammogram? It depends. Whether or not mammograms save enough lives to justify the expenditure depends on one's personal experience. What do you think would be the opinion of someone in whom such a cancer was picked up in a mammogram, treated in time, and cured?

Given these differences of opinion, many women are confused about whether or not to have regular mammograms.

Over the years, despite the occasional negative conclusion, most practicing doctors like me have stuck to their guns and continued to advise their patients to be routinely screened. Seven landmark studies in the 1970s and 1980s found that mammography saves lives. Then, in 2000, came the bombshell. Researchers in Denmark looked at these data again and determined that most of them were flawed. When they put all the evidence together, they concluded that the annual mammogram does not, in fact, result in any significant reduction in the death rate from breast cancer. Mammography's detractors had a field day; its proponents were put on the defensive. And that's where the matter stood—until now.

HERE'S WHAT'S NEW • Scientists in the United States, Sweden, Britain, and Taiwan in the largest and most credible study ever done to evaluate the impact of routine mammography on survival compared the number of deaths from breast cancer diagnosed in the 20 years *before* mammogram screening became available with the number in the 20 years *after* its introduction. The research was based on the histories and treatment of 210,000 Swedish women ages 20 to 69. The researchers found that death from breast cancer dropped 44 percent in women who had routine mammography. Among those who refused mammograms during this time period there was only a 16 percent reduction in death from this disease (the decrease was presumably due to better treatment of the malignancy).

Researchers at New York's Memorial Sloan-Kettering Cancer Center have found that magnetic resonance imaging (MRI) can detect small breast cancers missed by a mammogram. They recommend that women at high risk undergo *both* types of screening. (High-risk women are defined as those who have previously been treated for breast cancer, have a close relative such as a mother or sister with the disease, have tested positive for *mutations* in the BRCA1 or BRCA2 genes, or have benign breast lumps that could later cause cancer.)

Shortly after the appearance of the Denmark study, the American Cancer Society (ACS) issued its own mammogram guidelines in *A Cancer Journal for Clinicians* (Vol. 53, No. 3), making no major changes to its previous recommendations from 1997. The ACS also recommends breast ultrasound, MRI, or both for those at special risk for breast cancer. This organization emphasizes that between ages 20 and 39, women should make sure their doctor performs a manual breast examination at least every 3 years. It continues to endorse annual mammography between ages 40 and 69, except for women who have other serious health problems or a short life expectancy. The problem with mammograms in the 40-to-49 age group is the relatively high number of false-positives, especially in patients with dense breasts.

What about mammography after age 69? I still recommend it to my own patients, but many doctors aren't sure. Given the shortened life expectancy and higher risk of death from causes other than breast cancer, they conclude that mammography after age 69 may not be worthwhile. Some research suggests that bone mineral density can be used to predict the usefulness of mammograms for older women. Because high bone mineral density reflects higher estrogen levels throughout life, it may predict increased breast cancer risk. When researchers assessed the benefits of screening women age 70 and up, they found that mammograms in those with high bone mineral density would prevent 9.4 cancer deaths in every 10,000 women. Screening women with low bone mineral density would prevent only 1.4 additional deaths per 10,000 women. I present the facts to women in my practice and let them decide whether to continue having mammograms in their seventies.

The American Cancer Society is much less positive than it used to be about breast self-examination (BSE). However, I continue to make sure my patients know how to examine their breasts and that they do so regularly. Over the years, a few of them have detected tumors between their regularly scheduled mammograms or office visits.

THE BOTTOM LINE • Routine mammograms are important, especially for women between ages 50 and 69. In my own practice, I recommend one every 3 years to all female patients, starting at age 40 and annually thereafter. However, it's important to have a mammogram every year if you're at high risk or have a benign breast tumor.

Women whose breasts are dense should have a sonogram as well as a mammogram to clarify the significance of "suspicious" lumps. The latest research indicates that MRIs are especially useful in high-risk women and reduce the chance of missing a small cancer. It may be wise to have both a mammogram and an MRI if you're at high risk. Given the high cost of MRIs, discuss with your doctor whether just a sonogram (which is much less expensive) without the MRI might provide the answer.

With regard to breast self-examinations, I tell my patients to do them but not to be consumed by guilt if they miss them once in a while. ◦

CERVICAL CANCER

· · · · · · · · ·

What's the Optimal Screening Interval?

A PAP TEST is the most reliable way to detect the early stages of cervical cancer, a malignancy that strikes some 12,000 American women and causes about 4,100 deaths every year, according to the American Cancer Society (ACS). The test involves inserting a sterile metal or plastic instrument called a speculum into the vagina to separate the vaginal walls and expose the cervix. The cells are obtained from the cervix with a tiny brush or a small spatula and then examined for abnormalities under a microscope.

For years, the ACS recommended a Pap test every year. To ensure cost-effectiveness, lawmakers and insurance companies continually scrutinize the need for annual screening recommendations in healthy men and women and what intervals are optimal. Because of the low risk of developing cervical cancer, policymakers have been considering whether or not to extend the screening interval for cervical cancer to every 2 to 3 years.

HERE'S WHAT'S NEW

The ACS and the U.S. Preventive Services Task Force (USPSTF) both have issued a new set of guidelines for cervical cancer screening. They agree that it should begin to be done annually about 3 years after the onset of sexual activity or at age 21, whichever comes first. (Previous guidelines recommended starting screening at age 18.) At age 30, women who have had three consecutive normal Pap tests may wait 2 to 3 years before having another. They made this new recommendation because cervical cancer grows slowly and can still be cured even if not detected immediately. Also, more frequent screening, in addition to the anxiety it induces, can result in unnecessary biopsies and other procedures.

The new guidelines also suggest that the Pap test be discontinued at age 65 (it used to be age 70) in women who have not had an abnormal Pap test result any time during the preceding 10 years, except with HIV or a history of cervical cancer. They should continue to be tested.

The guidelines for women younger than 65 are supported by a large study of women age 30 to 64 reported in the October 16, 2003 issue of *The New England Journal of Medicine*. Testing every 3 years resulted in an average excess risk of cervical cancer in only three cases in 100,000.

However, researchers at Kaiser Permanente health maintenance organization reviewed the history of 1,416 of their patients, 482 of whom had cervical cancer, and concluded that the risk of missing an early diagnosis of cervical cancer doubles if a woman is screened at 2-to-3-year intervals, instead of once a year.

THE BOTTOM LINE

I suggest a compromise. If you're not at special risk, extend the screening interval to three years. But stay with annual testing if you have had questionable findings in the past, or have any problem that compromises your immune system and makes you more vulnerable to cancer.

There's Something Better Than Just a Pap Test

I WAS SURPRISED when some of my medical students didn't know what the "Pap" in Pap test stands for. Pap is neither an instrument nor a chemical. It's an abbreviation for the tongue-twisting name George Papanicolaou, the doctor who devised the test. My students' lack of awareness is especially surprising not only because the Pap test is one of the most important techniques used in medicine but also because Dr. Papanicolaou did his work at *their* medical school, Weill Cornell Medical College. More than that, his bust sits in the entrance hall through which they pass several times a day! (I try to teach them to be more observant doctors than they are students.)

The Pap test remains the best way to detect the earliest precancerous cell changes in the cervix. "Cell abnormalities" often reported generate ongoing anxiety, especially when follow-up tests or treatments are recommended for months or even years. Until recently, if needed to be repeated every few months to make sure that any suspicious cells cleared up or began to look more like cancer.

Not every "abnormal"-looking cell is destined to become malignant. In a study of almost 350,000 women who underwent routine Pap testing, British researchers found in follow-up that 80 percent never developed cancer! These numbers should reassure women that "cell abnormalities" are not a death sentence.

Identifying a woman's previous infection with the human papillomavirus (HPV) also can reduce the need for repeated testing. There are close to 100 strains of HPV, and they cause various problems, including warts (benign noncancerous tumors) in the genital area and elsewhere. Roughly 30 of these strains are spread through sexual contact and they infect an estimated 20 percent of sexually active women in the United States. (Some 50 to 75 percent of sexually active adults will have been infected at some point in their lives.)

Although HPV infection commonly does not result in long-term health problems, some infected women do go on to develop cervical cancer. Indeed, most patients with cervical cancer test positive for HPV antibodies. This means that if you have a "suspicious" Pap test result but test *negative* for HPV, you're at little risk for cervical cancer. You should still have a follow-up exam, but less frequently and with much less anxiety. The obvious conclusion is that there is much to be said (other than the cost) for getting an HPV test at the same time that you have your Pap smear.

HERE'S WHAT'S NEW

The FDA has approved a new screening method for cervical cancer that does just that. It combines a Pap test with one that can detect the DNA of the 13 strains of HPV linked with 99 percent of cervical cancers. The Pap test alone is only 70 to 80 percent sensitive in detecting cervical cancer; other HPV testing is 85 to 95 percent reliable. By comparison, the combined test, called the DNAwithPap and developed by the Digene Corporation, the accuracy is shown to be 97.8 percent. A negative DNAwithPap result is a virtual guarantee that you do not have cervical cancer. What's more, you're unlikely to develop it (unless, of course, you become infected with HPV at a later date). Preliminary guidelines from the ACS state that a woman who has a negative DNAwithPap result may wait 3 years before having another test. I agree with that recommendation.

In other relevant news about cervical cancer, researchers at the National Cancer Institute believe that long-term use of birth control pills increases the risk of cervical cancer in women who have HPV. Such women should have both a Pap test and an HPV test, or the recently approved DNAwithPap.

THE BOTTOM LINE

You may continue to have regular Pap tests as recommended, but for peace of mind, I suggest the new DNAwithPap test that also looks for evidence of the dangerous HPV infection. It's almost 98 percent accurate. Although it costs between $50 and $60 and some insurers won't pay for it, it needs to be done only every 3 years, and you can skip the annual Pap test.

New Hope for Cervical Cancer Survivors Who Want a Family

IF A ROUTINE PAP TEST reveals definite evidence of cervical cancer, and you've had these screens regularly, chances are the disease is at Stage 1 and early enough to cure. But don't panic! Over 50 percent of the 12,000 such cancers diagnosed every year in this country are Stage 1, and 92 percent of them can be cured.

The best treatment for such a malignancy is removal of the cancer—lock, stock, and barrel. In the past, that almost always meant taking out not only the cancerous cervix but the entire uterus as well—in short, a uterectomy. But that means no more babies, obviously devastating to a woman of childbearing age who has not yet started or completed her family.

An alternative to the uterectomy is the radical trachelectomy, which preserves a portion of healthy cervix, along with an opening large enough to allow normal menstrual flow. The uterus is left intact. The cervical stump can support the weight of a growing fetus that will be delivered by Cesarean section. However, this more limited operation is generally only offered to women with the earliest stages of cervical cancer.

HERE'S WHAT'S NEW

Doctors at the Albert Einstein College of Medicine in New York City reported to the Annual Clinical Meeting of the American College of Obstetricians and Gynecologists their experience with 32 women with early cervical cancer. All of the patients who underwent the procedure that left the uterus behind had normal periods within the next 3 months, and two of them subsequently delivered normal babies. None had evidence of recurrence of the cancer.

THE BOTTOM LINE

If you are of childbearing age and want to have a child but have been diagnosed with Stage 1 cervical cancer, ask your gynecologist whether you are a candidate for a radical trachelectomy, instead of the traditional uterectomy. Women in whom only the cancer is removed, leaving a portion of cervix and the uterus behind, remain fertile. After a 2-year wait, they can become pregnant and have the child by Cesarean section. It's important for this message to reach women with early cervical cancer who want to have or continue to bear children.

CHILDBIRTH COMPLICATIONS

· · · · · · · · ·

Deliver a Healthy Infant

As MANY AS 25 PERCENT of pregnant women harbor a bacterium known as Group B streptococcus (GBS). Because it may produce no symptoms other than occasional mild urinary complaints, the infection sometimes goes undiagnosed and untreated. (Don't confuse Group B with Group A streptococcus, which typically causes a bad sore throat.)

Although GBS usually doesn't harm the mother, it can be dangerous to her infant who contracts it while passing through the birth canal. In fact, GBS is the most common life-threatening infection of newborns in the United States and a leading cause of their death. Every year, in this country alone, GBS affects more than 1,600 babies at birth. One in 20 of them dies, and those who survive may be left with chronic problems such as poor hearing or vision, learning disabilities, or other neurological disorders.

HERE'S WHAT'S NEW

The American College of Obstetricians and Gynecologists now recommends that all pregnant women be screened routinely for GBS with vaginal and rectal swabs between the 35th and 37th weeks of pregnancy. The FDA recently has approved a new, faster test that identifies the infection in an hour. (It used to take up to 2 days.) This earlier result will protect the infants of infected women who can then be given intravenous doses of the appropriate antibiotic during labor and before delivery in time to prevent the transmission of GBS to their infant.

THE BOTTOM LINE

If you're pregnant, regardless of whether you have symptoms of genitourinary infection, you should be screened in the weeks before your delivery to make sure you are not harboring Group B streptococcus. Most doctors do this testing, but ask yours anyway just to be sure. Unfortunately, a few infants become infected despite this therapy, so ask your pediatrician about the warning signs and symptoms of GBS infection (such as pneumonia and meningitis) in the first days of life.

Wait! Prevent Premature Delivery

PRETERM DELIVERY (when the baby is born before the 37th week of pregnancy) is the most important problem facing obstetricians and pregnant women today. Worldwide, more than 13 million babies are born prematurely every year, and the incidence is rising. In the United States, one out of eight babies is born too soon.

The consequences of premature delivery range from stillbirth (especially before 30 weeks) to disabilities later in life that include learning delays, cerebral palsy, blindness, and deafness. Even babies born only 2 to 4 weeks premature can experience significant delays in their development, something every woman considering early Cesarean section for nonmedical reasons should bear in mind. Let nature take its course unless there is some compelling health reason to have a preterm Cesarean.

Women at greatest risk for premature labor (1) have a history of previous premature births; (2) are pregnant with twins, triplets, or more; (3) have a less than 6-month gap between pregnancies; or (4) are troubled by chronic uterine or vaginal infections. Other known risk factors that should be controlled include:

- Nutritional deficiencies and consumption of junk food during pregnancy
- Use of alcohol, tobacco, and illicit drugs
- High blood pressure
- Chronic gum disease

Unfortunately, the uterus for no apparent reason sometimes begins contracting before it should, and the baby is born too soon. Doctors don't always know why this happens, and most of the drugs given to prevent premature labor don't really work. When they do, it's only for a day or two. Bed rest, the old standby, is also usually not effective.

HERE'S WHAT'S NEW

Researchers in Denmark have come up with a fascinating and important observation regarding premature births. They analyzed the obstetrical history of more than 8,000 pregnant women, asking each one how much fish they regularly ate during pregnancy. They found that the more fish eaten, the lower the risk of premature birth—7 percent among those who consumed no fish at all, but only 2 percent in women who ate it once a week!

What is it about fish that offers this protection? It's docosahexanoic acid (DHA), one of the omega-3 fatty acids present in oily fish such as mackerel, herring, trout, salmon, and sardines. DHA suppresses the formation of prostaglandins, chemicals that cause the pregnant uterus to contract and are used to stimulate the onset of labor.

Scientists at Wake Forest University in Winston-Salem, North Carolina and 19 other research centers have come up with another important finding of their own. They studied a group of women who had previously delivered at least one baby before 37 weeks. They gave these women either a placebo or weekly injections of the drug 17-alpha-hydroxyprogesterone caproate (17P), a synthetic form of the hormone progesterone starting between 16 and 20 weeks into pregnancy and until the 36th week. Progesterone levels in the blood normally begin to rise early in pregnancy and continue to do so throughout its course. This hormone relaxes the smooth muscle of the uterus and makes it less able to contract. At the same time, it builds up the uterine lining and placenta to provide nutrition for the embryo and stimulates the breast glands in preparation for breastfeeding.

The results of this study were very impressive. Women treated with 17P were 42 percent less likely to deliver before 32 weeks and had 34 percent fewer deliveries before 37 weeks than those on placebo. What's more, the incidence of complications among the newborns was also less in the women who had received the drug. The FDA currently approves 17P only for the treatment of infertility, not for preventing premature births. If further studies document these findings, I'm sure that will change.

A pregnant woman's dental health also determines when she will deliver her baby. When researchers at the University of Alabama treated gum infections in 366 pregnant women before their 35th week by scaling and root planing (but not antibiotics), there was an 84 percent reduction of premature births.

THE BOTTOM LINE

If you have a history of giving birth prematurely or are vulnerable to doing so because of the risk factors previously listed, insist on attentive prenatal care. See your obstetrician regularly, get lots of rest, eat a well-balanced diet, and take all the prenatal vitamins that have been prescribed. Also have your dentist check your mouth for evidence of gum disease. It's not always apparent, and I don't know any obstetricians who check the teeth, so you have to ask. Cleaning the teeth and correcting periodontal disease can significantly reduce your risk of going into premature labor. In addition, eat one serving of fish every week or take omega-3 fatty acids in capsule form. Avoid tuna, mackerel, tilefish, swordfish, and shark because of their high mercury content (although canned light tuna is safe). Finally, ask your doctor whether the FDA has already approved weekly 17P injections between the 16th and 20th weeks of pregnancy for women at high risk for premature labor.

CHRONIC FATIGUE
SYNDROME

● ● ● ● ● ● ● ● ●

Tired of Being Tired

DESPITE ALL THE FANCY time- and energy-saving devices in modern society and the fact that fewer among us actually "labor" for a living anymore, the most common complaint I hear from adults of both genders is surprisingly: "Why am I so tired?"

Most healthy people feel "wiped out" now and then—usually for an obvious reason such as lack of sleep, perhaps because of a large prostate that has nature calling them too often during the night, or a hangover, anxiety, depression, or jet lag. Once the cause is identified and corrected, their normal energy returns. For some people, however, fatigue lingers and lingers. And doctors aren't always sure what to do about it—or why it happens.

If you remain exhausted day in, day out, for weeks on end for no apparent reason, no matter how much you rest or how long you sleep, your body is telling you that something is wrong. Don't ignore that signal! There are many possible reasons for the way you feel, and a careful, thorough workup will almost always reveal the source of your problem.

Your doctor will likely test you for everything from viruses and hypoglycemia to candida and allergies, and sometimes your results are all normal. The scenario of a severely and chronically tired patient testing normal for "everything" is so common that in 1988, some U.S. doctors decided to give it a name—chronic fatigue syndrome (CFS)—and designated it a "real" illness. However, many American-trained physicians are hesitant to name something they don't understand. Many would not accept CFS as a real diagnosis. I was one of them, but I've since changed my mind. I'm now convinced that CFS does exist and is probably due either to some derangement of the immune system, possibly triggered by an as-yet-unidentified virus; or it's an allergy; or the result of some hormonal imbalance. Despite the dissenters, the medical establishment officially legitimized CFS in 1993, although its cause or causes remain a mystery.

Although there are no reliable statistics concerning the incidence of CFS, I suspect that hundreds of thousands of Americans suffer from it. It can strike anyone at any age, but is two to four times more common in women of childbearing age, most of whom are white and middle-income.

CFS often sets in after an infection such as the flu, a stomach virus, or a bout of diarrhea. In some patients it follows an emotional crisis.

The formal criteria for the diagnosis of CFS are as follows:

- Fatigue that persists or recurs for at least six months

- The exclusion of any other condition that might account for the fatigue

- The distinct onset over a period of hours or days of at least four of the following symptoms that continue for at least 6 months: severe exhaustion, low-grade fever, sore throat, painful lymph nodes, generalized muscle weakness and aches, prolonged fatigue after exercise, joint pains, generalized headaches, disturbed sleep, and nervous system complaints such as memory loss, inability to concentrate, and irritability

HERE'S WHAT'S NEW

Despite what you read on the Internet, there is no proven or secret remedy for CFS, nor is there much new on its treatment. Some patients recover completely within 5 years, while others get better for a while and then relapse in cycles.

If you suffer from CFS, your best course of action is to stick with some of the following tried-and-true guidelines that may alleviate your symptoms:

- Eliminate any food or medication to which you are allergic.

- Avoid any activity that tires you, but continue to perform the gentle home-based exercises prescribed by your doctor or a qualified physiotherapist.

- If you have flu-like symptoms (headache, low-grade fever, joint and muscle aches) take aspirin, Tylenol, or a nonsteroidal anti-inflammatory drug (NSAID).

- Consider taking an antidepressant. It may improve sleep and reduce fatigue and muscle pain.

- Ask your doctor about Tagamet (cimetidine), an antiulcer drug, which can strengthen the immune system. This therapy is still experimental.

- Consider intravenous gamma globulin, which has been tried with questionable success but is worth looking into.

- Eat "healthy." This is no time for fad diets. Emphasize whole grains, beans, rice, fish, and fresh fruits and vegetables; take it easy on alcohol and high-fat foods. I advise my patients to consume liberal amounts of garlic (either fresh cloves or as a commercial extract), because garlic is said to stimulate the immune system. There is no proof that it does so, but it can't hurt to take it.

Since conventional medicine has so little to offer in the way of specific treatment for CFS, there are several alternative approaches you may try (but let your doctor know you're doing so). For example, acupuncture and acupressure are said to be successful in some cases. There's no harm in trying them. Also, various herbs have been reported to improve CFS, but the evidence is anecdotal. The most popular ones are echinacea, goldenseal, milk thistle, and ginseng. Chinese herbalists have their own concoctions that they say help. Try them if you're desperate. Finally, I recommend certain mind-body approaches such as tai chi, meditation, relaxation, guided imagery, qigong, and yoga that increase your energy level by reducing stress.

THE BOTTOM LINE

Chronic fatigue syndrome is a real disease whose cause is unknown and for which no specific treatment exists. As a result, many insurance companies refuse to pay for its care. Although the medical establishment has formally listed the criteria for diagnosing CFS, it remains a diagnosis of exclusion. That means that every other possible cause of the profound fatigue and other symptoms described above must be ruled out. If your doctor is unable to reach a diagnosis or does not believe that CFS is a real condition, get a second opinion by another physician. Once the CFS diagnosis is made, try the therapies previously listed.

COLD AND FLU

· · · · · · · · ·

Echinacea—Is It All It's Cracked Up to Be?

THOUSANDS OF CONSUMERS around the world believe that echinacea mobilizes infection-fighting white blood cells in the body and strengthens immune defenses, and therefore helps prevent the common cold and relieve its symptoms. Sales of echinacea account for 10 percent of the billions of dollars spent on herbal supplements in this country. We even keep echinacea in our home medicine cabinet, even though I am not convinced that it really works. But my wife is, so who am I to argue?

HERE'S WHAT'S NEW

Two research reports on echinacea about 3 months apart cast doubt on its effectiveness. Let me tell you about them so you can decide for yourself whether it's worth taking.

In the first study, reported in the *Annals of Internal Medicine*, doctors at the University of Wisconsin evaluated the effect of echinacea on 148 students who came down with the common cold. In this controlled study, half the students received the herb and the rest were given a placebo. Neither the doctors nor the patients knew who was receiving what. When the results were analyzed, there was no real difference between the treated and placebo groups in terms of the severity of the cold or its duration. In fact, cold symptoms actually lasted a little longer in those receiving the herb. Proponents of echinacea say that these results don't mean much because the researchers used only one type of echinacea (*Echinacea angustifolia*) and their findings may not necessarily apply to other types.

The second paper raises even more doubts as to the wisdom of spending your hard-earned money on echinacea. It looked into the manufacturing process of this herb, given the fact that the FDA doesn't routinely monitor supplements, as it does prescription drugs. Doctors at Presbyterian/St. Luke's Hospital Medical Center in Denver analyzed the contents of echinacea-labeled products sold in retail stores in the Denver area. Among the 59 preparations sampled (21 of which claimed to be standardized, meaning that there is no variation from bottle to bottle), 52 percent contained the ingredients as labeled. A full 10 percent contained no echinacea at all! What's more, among those claiming to be standardized, only 43 percent actually were. All in all, a rather poor showing.

THE BOTTOM LINE

If you take echinacea to treat (or prevent) your common cold and you think it works for you, by all means continue to use it, especially if it agrees with you. So what if the benefit you perceive is all in your head? You feel better, don't you? But if you've never been convinced that the herb is effective, yet you continue to spend money on it because everyone (including your wife) tells you it works, use this information as the justification for trying something else, such as chicken soup.

Here's an afterthought suggested by my echinacea-hooked wife. She asks, "What if the echinacea preparation that was tested in the first study and found to be ineffective was among the 10 percent that didn't contain the active ingredient? In that case, concluding that echinacea doesn't work isn't really justified, is it?" That's a far-fetched possibility, but who ever would have thought of it—except my wife?

Flu Treatments—New and Old

EVERY YEAR, MORE THAN 100,000 people are hospitalized because of the flu, and 36,000 of them die. Most have not been vaccinated and are older than age 65. The vaccine protects 70 to 90 percent of healthy adults against the flu and prevents it from developing into pneumonia in 50 to 60 percent of the elderly and those with compromised immune systems.

Here are two basic facts you need to know about the flu: (1) Almost everybody should get the flu vaccine. (2) The flu is not caused by a bacterium, so antibiotics won't make you better.

Years ago the flu vaccine was recommended only for the elderly and the chronically sick. However, most doctors now feel that everyone should be protected against its ravages.

Flu treatment has always consisted basically of reducing the severity of its signs and symptoms—fever, cough, aches, and pains. Take Tylenol (acetaminophen) or Advil (ibuprofen), cough suppressants, and lots of fluids. And don't forget bed rest.

Several anti-flu medications, aimed both at prevention and treatment, were introduced a few years ago. The older ones are Symmetrel (amantadine) and its newer, preferred derivative Flumadine (rimantadine). These pills typically are taken at the earliest onset of symptoms.

Also, if for some reason you can't or won't have the vaccine and have been exposed to the flu, the amantadine family of drugs helps reduce your risk of becoming infected. (They only work against type A flu, not type B.)

Newer medications actually attack the flu virus itself and prevent it from reproducing. One medication, Relenza (zanamivir), is inhaled orally; the other, Tamiflu (oseltamivir), comes in pill form. Both shorten the duration of the infection and reduce the severity of its symptoms. Tamiflu also is approved for *preventing* flu types A and B in those ages 13 or older.

HERE'S WHAT'S NEW

Elderberry has been used for centuries to treat everything from respiratory tract infections to gastrointestinal symptoms to depression. In fact, it has been called the "medicine chest of the common people."

Now comes word from researchers at the University of Oslo School of Medicine in Norway that an extract from the black elderberry reduces the symptoms and duration of flu types A and B. Flu patients given this herbal extract recovered in about 3 days as compared to 7 days in those taking a placebo. Apparently, some ingredient in elderberry attacks the flu virus and prevents it from attaching to the body's cells and making us sick.

The specific preparation used in this study was developed by an Israeli virologist and is marketed as Sambucol. It may not yet be available in this form in the United States, but ask your health food store if they sell other elderberry preparations. It may be worth trying (along with the conventional medications) if you come down with the flu.

THE BOTTOM LINE

Although several medications minimize the severity and duration of the flu, there is no cure. You may want to consider taking black elderberry extract, which has recently been shown to be an effective palliative for this infection as soon as the diagnosis is confirmed. But use it along with the proven antiviral agents now available for this infection.

More Flu Shots, Less Death

I'M ALWAYS AMAZED that so many of my patients resist getting an annual flu shot. These are the same people who clamor for MRIs, CT scans, colonoscopies, and other time-consuming, expensive, unpleasant procedures, yet balk at a little jab in the arm once a year. (Don't get me wrong, these other tests are important, especially the colonoscopy, but it's often easier to "sell" them than it is a flu shot.)

Some of the reasons for rejection are:

A. "I had one last year."

B. "No, sir, never again. I got the flu after the last shot."

C. "Look, doc, I never get the flu."

D. "I'll take it only if I get the flu."

E. "I can't take it because I am allergic to eggs and chicken."

Here's how I respond to each of these excuses:

A. Unlike other vaccinations, such as the one against pneumonia, which lasts for years and usually need not be taken again after age 65, a new formulation of flu vaccine is made annually because the specific flu virus changes from year to year. Last year's supply won't protect you.

B. The flu vaccine contains the dead virus. It cannot cause the flu. If you come down with the infection after you were vaccinated, it's because you were already harboring the bug, and it takes about 2 weeks for the vaccine to work.

C. Everybody is vulnerable to the flu. If you have never had it, it's probably only a matter of time until you will—unless you get the shot.

D. Once you come down with the symptoms, it's too late for the vaccine to work (although now some effective antiviral drugs can reduce the duration of the illness and the severity of its symptoms).

E. Having an allergy to eggs or chicken is the only valid reason not to have the shot.

HERE'S WHAT'S NEW

The Veterans Affairs Medical Center in Minneapolis, Minnesota, compiled data from 280,000 men and women 65 years and older during flu season in 1998, 1999, and 2000. Those who received a flu shot not only had a 29 to 32 percent lower incidence of pneumonia and flu but also were 19 percent less likely to be hospitalized for heart disease and had 16 to 23 percent fewer hospital admissions for stroke. Overall, a flu shot reduced the risk of dying of any cause by 48 to 50 percent. I wonder if reading these impressive figures will have any impact on all the naysayers in my practice.

Here's more good news. If you're between ages 5 and 49, you can now be vaccinated with a nasal spray, recently approved by the FDA. No more needles!

Now for some bad news. It seems that the flu vaccine is not quite as effective as we used to think, especially for the elderly. Men and women older than age 80 are many more times likely to develop influenza even after being vaccinated than those 15 to 20 years younger. That's probably because their immune systems are unable to respond to the vaccine and so don't produce enough antibodies to ward off the infection. The practical implications of this observation are that if you are older and were given the vaccine but develop what appears to be the flu, see your doctor about it. Don't assume that it's only a cold simply because you were vaccinated.

THE BOTTOM LINE

The flu vaccine remains the number one safeguard against the flu. Young or old, healthy or sick, get vaccinated—but not if you're allergic to eggs or chicken. And if you're between ages 5 and 49, you can have the vaccine as a nasal spray.

No Aspirin for Kids under Age 16

FOR YEARS, doctors have been warning parents not to give their children aspirin because of a rare disorder called Reye's syndrome, which for some unknown reason can develop in children (and occasionally in adults) who have taken aspirin to relieve symptoms of a recent respiratory viral infection or chickenpox. Although Reye's syndrome occurs in only one in a million cases, when it does strike, it can be fatal. It attacks the brain and liver, and unless diagnosed early, it causes death within a few days. There is no cure for Reye's. Treatment consists of reducing the elevated pressure the disease causes in the brain.

HERE'S WHAT'S NEW

Since 1986, the United Kingdom has reduced the incidence of Reye's by banning the use of aspirin for anyone younger than age 12. The U.K.'s Medicines Control Agency has now expanded the limit to age 16 because of the Reye's-related death of a 13-year-old who is thought to have taken aspirin.

THE BOTTOM LINE

Do not give aspirin to any child younger than age 16. Use Tylenol instead.

WHAT THE DOCTOR ORDERED?

SHOULD YOU BOTHER TAKING COUGH MEDICINE?

• The two medications most people ask for when they have a cold or the flu are antibiotics and cough medicine. Doctors now know better than to prescribe antibiotics at the drop of a hat like they once did. That's because most upper-respiratory infections are due to a virus against which antibiotics are useless. Taking them only increases your likelihood of becoming resistant to them, and then when you really need them in the future, they don't work.

Cough medicines are another matter. They usually contain two kinds of ingredients, one to loosen respiratory congestion (an expectorant) and the other to suppress the cough. Surely there isn't any harm in taking them—or is there?

HERE'S WHAT'S NEW • Representatives of the American College of Physicians–American Society of Internal Medicine, a group that represents more than 100,000 doctors, have concluded that cough syrups are usually a waste of money. There is little or no evidence that the expectorants they contain benefit upper- or lower-respiratory tract infections (despite the manufacturers' insistence to the contrary). If you need to loosen mucus, the best way to do it probably is to drink more fluids.

What about something to stop the cough? Most suppressants contain codeine or one of its derivatives, and they do stop a dry, irritating cough. The downside is their side effects, such as constipation and drowsiness. If your cough is loose, it's not a good idea to suppress it, because the cough is nature's way of getting rid of the phlegm.

THE BOTTOM LINE • There is some disagreement about these recommendations. Expectorants probably don't do much good, although everyone agrees that they can do no harm. As for suppressants, I think that if a dry, hacking cough is interfering with your sleep, you should take cough syrup. However, if the cough is already loose, a suppressant will prevent you from getting rid of annoying mucus in your respiratory tract. Try the other time-honored alternatives first, such as hot beverages and chicken soup, and keep the cough syrup handy just in case. If you weaken and do take a couple of teaspoons, don't worry about it. Just make sure you have a laxative handy and be prepared to feel a little drowsy. •

COLON CANCER

. . . .

Fiber *Does* Protect Against Colon Cancer

ABOUT 30 YEARS AGO, a British doctor named Denis Burkitt, working in Africa, made three interesting observations about the poor people living there: (a) they produced more feces than those in developed countries, (b) they ate much more fiber, and (c) they had a much lower incidence of colon cancer. He put these facts together and came up with the hypothesis that fiber in the diet protects against constipation and cancer of the bowel. The mechanism he suggested to explain fiber's beneficial effect is that it dilutes and binds cancer-causing agents and adds bulk to the stool, so these carcinogens are excreted more quickly. According to another theory, fiber decreases the quantity of bile acids excreted by the liver thus reducing the irritation to the bowel walls. Whichever reason you believe, you end up with fewer instances of bowel cancer when you eat enough fiber.

For more than a quarter century, this relationship between fiber and bowel cancer remained dogma in this country. Breakfast food makers had a bonanza with it because grain (along with fruits and vegetables) is a major source of dietary fiber. Then in 1999, findings in the ongoing Nurses Study at Harvard, the source of many important epidemiological observations, apparently debunked the fiber-cancer link. Follow-up of more than 88,000 women over a 16-year period revealed that the incidence of colon cancer was not affected by the amount of fiber they consumed. The following year, two other studies conducted over a 4-year period also failed to demonstrate any correlation between cancer and diets or supplements high in fiber. The theory linking fiber and cancer has remained in limbo—until now.

HERE'S WHAT'S NEW

According to two major new studies published in *The Lancet* medical journal, one done in the United States and the other in Europe, the amount of fiber you consume makes a *big* difference in your vulnerability to colon cancer. The average daily fiber consumption in this country is about 16 grams a day; compared to 22 grams a day in Europe. (Here's what this means in practical terms: one slice of whole wheat bread contains 2 grams of fiber, a banana has 3 grams, an apple or a cup of brown rice contain 3.5 grams, a half cup of a fiber-rich cereal may have as much as 10 grams.)

The European research involved more than 500,000 people in 10 countries, dwarfing all earlier studies. Subjects who ate 35 grams of fiber a day had a 40 percent lower rate of bowel cancer than those who consumed only 15 grams a day. In the United States, the impact of fiber was evaluated among 3,600 men and women who'd previously had colon polyps (which often are precursors of cancer) and compared their outcome with that of about 34,000 healthy individuals. Those who ate the most fiber (36 grams a day) had a 27 percent lower incidence of colon cancer than those who ate the least (12 grams a day).

THE BOTTOM LINE

Any way you look at it, there is no downside to eating lots of fiber. It helps control weight; it makes for softer, more comfortable stools; and most important, it reduces the risk of colon cancer. Seems like a no-brainer to me. So, do yourself a favor, and enjoy a cup of a high-fiber grain cereal in the morning. Just be sure that if you increase your fiber intake that you do it gradually and drink lots of water, too.

Don't Blush, Look Before You Flush!

COLON CANCER is a major killer, but it can be cured if it's detected early enough. Everyone should have a routine colonoscopy starting at age 50. If nothing is found, the test should be repeated in 10 years; however, if polyps are detected in your initial colonoscopy or you have a strong family history of this malignancy, the colonoscopy should be done every 3 years. Remember, however, that between tests it's important to report to your doctor any new abdominal complaints—changes in bowel habits, or the appearance of blood in your stool. Blood in the stool is not always visible, so ask for a fecal occult blood test, a little card on which you place a stool specimen to be analyzed for blood.

It's also a good idea to look at your own stool after every bowel movement. That's what the British medical establishment wants everyone to do, and to encourage people to do so, they've come up with the slogan, "Don't Blush, Look Before You Flush."

HERE'S WHAT'S NEW

British gastroenterologists have pointed out a surprising problem with this advice—the use of toilet disinfectants, most of which are bright blue. These solutions make it more difficult to tell if there's blood in the stool. So they have embarked on a campaign in the United Kingdom to discourage manufacturers from coloring their toilet disinfectants. We should, too.

THE BOTTOM LINE

I suggest you stop using colored toilet disinfectants. Instead, look carefully at the stool and the color of the water in the toilet bowl to detect the presence of blood. It can save your life.

Prevent Colon Cancer from Recurring— Or Ever Happening

SUPPOSE YOU'RE A CANCER SURVIVOR, one of the lucky ones. Your colon (or colorectal) cancer was discovered in time and removed. But you aren't free and clear because you know you're more likely to develop cancer again, there or elsewhere, than someone who's never had the problem. This is true especially if you developed the cancer before you turned 60 or if you also have chronic inflammatory bowel disease. So your doctor has advised you to have another colonoscopy in a year, looking not only for a recurrence of the cancer itself, but for the presence of new polyps that sometimes become malignant later on. You were told also to look carefully at every stool you produce for evidence of blood.

There's lots more you can do to reduce the risk of another colorectal cancer. For starters, eat less red meat and have at least five to seven servings a day of fruits and vegetables, as well as other foods from plant sources (beans, grain products, and pasta). Exercise regularly, too, and don't just watch your weight, do something about it if you're too heavy. You may think that smoking is bad for only the lungs. The fact is smokers are 30 to 40 percent more likely to die of colon cancer than nonsmokers. Finally, because booze is a risk factor for bowel cancer, limit your intake to one or two drinks per day.

You were lucky the first time around. Don't tempt fate now by failing to heed this advice—as well as what follows.

HERE'S WHAT'S NEW

Researchers at the University of North Carolina in Chapel Hill studied 635 subjects with a history of colorectal cancer. They found that those who took an adult dose of aspirin (325 milligrams) every day had a 35 percent lower risk of developing colon polyps than subjects given a placebo. That's important because although only 5 to 10 percent of colon polyps become cancerous in individuals with no previous history, that risk is greatly increased if you've previously had a malignancy of the colon. Other studies have shown that nonsteroidal anti-inflammatories (NSAIDs) also reduce the risk of colon cancer, presumably because of the same anti-inflammatory effect as aspirin.

And, there's even more you can do if you have a history of colon cancer. If, for any reason, you can't take aspirin (either because you're allergic to it or it makes you bleed from the stomach), ask your doctor about calcium supplements. They, too, can prevent polyp formation. Even if you have no problem with aspirin, take the calcium anyway— and protect your bones as well as your bowel!

Here's even more good news! This time it's tea, one of the most widely consumed and inexpensive beverages in the world. Studies funded by the National Cancer Institute have determined that drinking three cups of green or white tea every day can prevent certain colon cancers (black tea does not appear to be as protective). Researchers believe that the beneficial action of these types of tea stems from their polyphenol content. Tea is especially effective when combined with an anti-inflammatory drug.

THE BOTTOM LINE

Fortunately, there is a great deal you can do to prevent recurrence of colon cancer, and even its first appearance. Lifestyle and diet are important. Adding aspirin or one of the NSAIDs like Advil (ibuprofen) is important, as are calcium supplements and the daily consumption of green or white tea.

However, none of these steps is a substitute for regular screening—this includes annual screening of stool specimens for traces of blood not visible to the human eye. You should have a colonoscopy every year if you've already had a colon cancer.

For someone without a previous history of colon polyps or cancer, I recommend a colonoscopy at age 50 with follow-ups at appropriate intervals based on what was found and details of your family history. Routinely, your doctor should request a flexible sigmoidoscopy (a procedure that examines part of the colon) every 5 years and a colonoscopy (that looks at the entire colon) every 10 years.

WHAT THE DOCTOR ORDERED?

BETA-CAROTENE: GOOD AND BAD • Everyone knows that fruits and vegetable are good for the heart and that they also reduce the risk of cancer. Carotenes are considered to be prime among the many ingredients that afford these health benefits. There are several different kinds of carotenes, the best known of which is beta-carotene. It is extracted from fruits and vegetables and put into capsules either alone or combined with other vitamins. Presumably, the logic for doing so is that if fruits and vegetables are good for you, then high doses of one of their main ingredients should be, too.

This assumption led to a famous study in Finland in the 1990s. Its purpose was to see whether taking beta-carotene would reduce the incidence of lung cancer in heavy cigarette smokers. The research project looked at 29,000 male subjects who were randomly assigned to one of four regimens: (1) beta-carotene alone, (2) beta-carotene and vitamin E, (3) vitamin E alone, or (4) a placebo. Neither the researchers nor the participants in the study knew who was getting what. After 8 years, researchers evaluated the findings. Guess what? Those subjects who received the beta-carotene had an 18 percent *higher* incidence of lung cancer and an 8 percent higher death rate from all causes than the "unlucky" controls who did not.

That destroyed the myth of beta-carotene, at least in my mind, although it continued to be advertised as a health panacea and sold in health food stores everywhere.

HERE'S WHAT'S NEW • A 2003 study at the Dartmouth Medical School looked once more at the impact of beta-carotene on cancer. The new target was colon polyps (which sometimes lead to colorectal cancer). As was the case with lung cancer, the researchers found that participants who received the usual daily 25-milligram dose of beta-carotene *and who smoked cigarettes or had more than one alcoholic drink a day or both* were at *twice* the risk of developing recurrent adenomas (polyps) when compared with the controls.

But here's the big news. The beta-carotene actually *reduced* the risk of these polyps by 44 percent in *nonsmokers and nondrinkers*. There appears to be something in tobacco and alcohol that interacts unfavorably with beta-carotene.

THE BOTTOM LINE • Fruits and vegetables are good for you. All their ingredients *working together* guard your health against various diseases. However, the effect of any single component is unpredictable. Beta-carotene is a case in point. It seems from at least two studies that when this supplement is given to drinkers or smokers, it *increases* the risk of certain cancers; however it appears to protect against colon polyps in people who neither drink nor smoke.

So here's my advice. Eat all the whole fruits and vegetables you can—at least 6 to 8 servings a day. If you can't manage that, take a daily 25-milligram dose of beta-carotene, but only *if you neither drink nor smoke*. (Avoid it if you're a smoker or drinker, even a social one.) Also, remember that beta-carotene is present in many multivitamins, so look at the label on the bottle of the one you're taking. •

DEEP VEIN THROMBOSIS

• • • • • • • • •

Take Blood Thinners for How Long?

EACH YEAR, an estimated two million Americans develop deep vein thrombosis (DVT), in which one or more blood clots form in the veins deep inside the leg. Signs and symptoms of DVT include pain and swelling of the leg, distention of the superficial veins just under the skin, and reddish-blue discoloration and increased warmth of the skin.

You're vulnerable to DVT after age 60 (although it can occur at any age), and the risk increases as you get older. However, the greatest danger is being confined to bed for 3 or more days for any reason—for example, because of chronic illness, an injury, or surgery. Women who take the estrogen-containing birth control pill and also smoke;

and anyone with heart or lung failure or a genetic predisposition to clotting is also a candidate for DVT.

Other risk factors include obesity, varicose veins, history of a previous clot, certain congenital heart defects, and hormone replacement therapy in postmenopausal women. DVT also has been referred to as the "economy class syndrome" when it occurs after sitting for hours on a plane in a small seat with little legroom.

The list of risks is long, but if any of the above situations applies to you, suspect DVT if you develop unexplained pain or tenderness in your legs. Before the availability of modern, noninvasive imaging procedures, contrast venography was the gold standard for diagnosing DVT. Dye was injected into the leg veins, and x-rays were then taken to indicate the location and size of the blood clot. That's no longer the way to go. Today, doctors use either a duplex ultrasound or an MRI. (I prefer the MRI because it's more sensitive, especially for detecting thrombosis in the calf veins.) However, the problem with the MRI is its cost. Ultrasound, though useful for revealing vein problems in other areas of the leg, does not detect thrombosis in the calf as accurately.

DVT is a serious illness on two counts. If the clots are large enough, they can obstruct the veins so that blood backs up and causes the legs to swell. More important, the clots themselves can break up and their fragments can travel along the body's network of veins, ending up in the lungs and blocking one or more pulmonary arteries. This complication, called pulmonary embolism, is responsible for an estimated 60,000 deaths every year in the United States.

These deaths are preventable if the DVT is properly diagnosed and treated immediately. Unfortunately, the classic symptoms often go unrecognized, undetected, and not reported to the doctor.

So always think of a pulmonary embolism, especially if you have been diagnosed with DVT and you experience any of the following signs or symptoms: chest pain that is worse when you take a deep breath, the onset of a cough without any cold or flu symptoms, or the presence of blood in the sputum. These signs and symptoms should raise the red flag of a pulmonary embolism not only if you have obvious DVT but also if you've recently been on a long trip, had surgery, or been confined to bed for 3 days or more.

If you suspect a pulmonary embolism, ask for a ventilation perfusion scan (VQ) of your lungs. It's a noninvasive procedure specifically designed to detect pulmonary blood clots. Once the attack is over:

- Resume your normal activities gradually and don't get overtired.
- Get plenty of rest but don't spend too much time in bed.
- Postpone any travel plans that call for long plane flights or car trips.
- If you're taking birth control pills, discuss another form of contraception with your doctor.
- Stop smoking.
- Don't cross your legs when lying in bed or sitting.

DVT, with or without a pulmonary embolus, should be treated by "thinning" the blood with anticoagulants as soon as the diagnosis is made. Two drugs usually are started simultaneously: heparin and Coumadin (warfarin). Heparin acts immediately, is given by injection under the skin or into a vein, and usually needs to be continued for 5 to 7 days. Warfarin is administered orally, acts in a different way, and takes a few days to reach effective levels in the blood. After it does so, the heparin is stopped and the warfarin is continued alone.

HERE'S WHAT'S NEW

For years, doctors have debated how long to continue warfarin therapy in patients with DVT, pulmonary embolus, or both. Staying on this medication indefinitely requires checking your blood every few weeks to see that the "thinning" level is optimal, or as Goldilocks would have put it, "Neither too thick nor too thin, but just right." However, a greater drawback of long-term anticoagulant use is the danger of internal bleeding. Such bleeding can occur spontaneously or after an injury. The hazard is especially great in older people who are prone to falling, making them vulnerable to brain hemorrhage. Also, one has to be careful about taking warfarin along with other drugs, such as aspirin, any of the NSAIDs, and even such widely used herbs as garlic and ginkgo. These combinations can increase the risk of bleeding.

The question of how long to continue anticoagulation was addressed in an important study involving hundreds of patients with DVT. Here are its important conclusions and recommendations.

If you've had DVT with or without a pulmonary embolus, you should be treated with heparin and warfarin together immediately. The heparin should be continued for 5 to 7 days and the warfarin for anywhere between 6 and 12 months. If whatever caused the DVT is no longer active and you're no longer at risk for it acting up, you may then stop the warfarin as far as this particular episode of DVT is concerned. However, there is a 5 to 10 percent risk of another clot forming during the next 12 months. So try not expose yourself during that interval to any of the risk factors for DVT.

Beyond the first year after discontinuing the anticoagulants, the risk of clots recurring drops to only 1 to 2 percent per year. No matter how long you continue the warfarin after your DVT—5 years, 10 years, or even longer—once you stop it, you will still have this "catch-up" risk of 5 to 10 percent for 1 year. That's presumably because of the body's reaction to going off warfarin—a kind of rebound phenomenon.

Some people (and their doctors) will decide not to take the risk and will opt to continue to take the anticoagulant indefinitely. As long as you do so, you'll be protected against DVT and embolism. The downside of staying on the warfarin is the risk of bleeding and the fact that you have the same 5 to 10 percent chance for DVT whenever you stop the therapy. Strange, but true!

THE BOTTOM LINE

Treating DVT with anticoagulants immediately after it's diagnosed can prevent the potentially lethal complication of a blood clot to the lung. After the original risk factors that cause the DVT are no longer present, this anticoagulant therapy usually is discontinued at some point. There's a 5 to 10 percent chance of another DVT occurring during the following 12 months. After that, the risk drops to between 1 and 2 percent. If you have a chronic disorder, such as heart failure or serious lung disease, it makes sense to continue long-term warfarin therapy (just as you would for an artificial heart valve or chronic atrial fibrillation). Otherwise you may want to take your chances and discontinue the warfarin after 1 year.

DEPRESSION

. . . .

No One Is Immune

AS ANY COUNTRY SINGER WILL ATTEST, everyone gets the blues now and then. But for 30 million Americans, that occasional sadness is chronic. Depression afflicts twice as many women as men, rich and poor alike. Although it occurs more frequently in older people, children are also plagued by it, and suicide is the leading cause of death among teenagers and young adults in the United States.

There are two basic types of depression. In the first, there is some obvious reason for your melancholy, but you may be overreacting to it—and for too long. For example, you may have lost a loved one or are in the midst of a nasty divorce. Or your depression may be due to the most treatable of all reasons—a drug you're taking, anything from an antibiotic to a birth control pill to a blood pressure-lowering agent. A depression with such an identifiable cause is the best kind to have because most people eventually "snap out of it" with or without professional help.

The other kind of depression comes on for no apparent reason. You may be sitting on top of the world as far as everyone else is concerned, but for you, the future is bleak. You can see no light at the end of the tunnel—and you don't know why. This type of depression may be part of a cyclical manic-depressive disorder that's full of ups and downs. One day you're wildly stimulated and full of energy, as though you've won the mental lottery. But then your mood swings to the other end of the spectrum—you're so down that all you can think about is suicide.

Your depression isn't always obvious to others. Some people can hide the way they feel. But even if they appear to be functioning normally, their depression stifles spontaneity and creativity; it hurts relationships with family, friends, and coworkers. If it persists long enough, it almost inevitably causes physical symptoms such as weight loss or weight gain, a poor appetite or an insatiable one, fatigue, irritability, stomach problems, impotence and lack of libido, insomnia—you name it. If it's bad enough, you'll harbor suicidal thoughts or even try to end it all, as 16,000 people succeed in doing every year in the United States.

How do you know if you're seriously depressed and not just temporarily down in the dumps? According to the latest edition of the American Psychiatric Association's *Diagnostic and Statistical Manual*, you have a *major* depression if you've had any *four* of the following symptoms for at least 2 weeks:

- Either you have severe insomnia, tossing and turning all night, or you're sleeping all the time.

- Either you have no appetite or you can't stop eating.

- You have no interest in doing anything or seeing anybody.

- You feel worthless and guilty, and you know there's no hope for you.

- You have trouble concentrating, and you can't make decisions.

- Suicidal thoughts run through your mind, and you've even tried to end it all.

- You realize that you're sad, but you just can't snap out of it.

- You're pessimistic about your future.

- You've started writing things down because your memory has become so poor, even though you're not yet 50.

- You're not doing nearly as well as you used to at school or at work because none of it really interests you anymore.

- You don't enjoy anything anymore, not even sex.

- You're always too tired to do anything, even watch TV.

- You always seem to have a headache, bellyache, or backache.

- You're restless and irritable.

- You're drinking a lot and taking more tranquilizers than ever.

- You've developed a "what difference does it make?" attitude about almost everything.

- You can't be bothered with people, even old friends. Crowds bother you.

- You have rushed to make a will and have even been thinking about your funeral.

HERE'S WHAT'S NEW

Modern therapy for depression still includes several older antidepressants such as the monoamine oxidase (MAO) inhibitors and tricyclics (of which Elavil is the best known). I don't prescribe these as much as I used to because even though they are effective, they have more unpleasant side effects than the newer medications called selective serotonin reuptake inhibitors (SSRIs). Depressed people have less serotonin, a neurotransmitter, than those who are not depressed. SSRIs act by increasing the concentration of serotonin in the brain. The first and best known of the SSRIs is Prozac (fluoxetine). Although many patients do well with it, others prefer Paxil (paroxetine), Effexor (venlafaxine), or Celexa (citalopram), to name but a few. They all differ a little from one another. Work with your doctor to find the one that's right for you. Although the SSRIs are generally well tolerated, they all can reduce your sex drive, increase your appetite and weight (or cause nausea), and leave you constipated. They're potent medications that your doctor should prescribe and monitor, so don't run out and "borrow" one of them from a friend.

Adults aren't the only ones who take antidepressants. Overall, 6 percent of children and teenagers in the United States take medication for depression, attention-deficit hyperactivity disorder, and other behavioral and emotional problems. Many of the drugs, especially the antidepressants, are the same as those given to adults, but have not been approved by the FDA for children.

After reviewing all available data, the FDA now believes that there is enough evidence of Prozac's effectiveness to warrant its approval for treating depression in children older than age 7. However, parents of these children should know that Prozac can cause nausea, fatigue, dizziness, difficulty concentrating, and nervousness. And they should bear in mind an additional adverse effect unique to kids and teenagers: They may grow more slowly and gain less weight and it's not yet known whether they eventually catch up.

What's true for Prozac doesn't necessarily apply to other SSRIs. For example, the FDA has ruled that Paxil should not be taken by anyone younger than age 18 because it is associated with a possible increased risk of suicidal impulses.

THE BOTTOM LINE

If you're an adult and you're down in the dumps, see a doctor and get a complete physical. Be sure to rule out all physical diseases or reactions to medications before starting any treatment. Even if there is no physical basis for your sadness, an antidepressant may help.

Depressed children and teenagers may be treated with Prozac if their doctors believe the symptoms warrant doing so. Such therapy is safe, according to the FDA. But if your child is taking Prozac, make sure a pediatrician closely monitors his or her weight and growth.

WHAT THE DOCTOR ORDERED?

ANTIDEPRESSANTS—ANOTHER CAUSE OF UPPER GASTROINTESTINAL BLEEDING • As we get older, blood vessels in the stomach and, to a lesser extent, the small intestine, become more vulnerable to irritation and bleeding. That's why older people who regularly take aspirin and/or a nonsteroidal anti-inflammatory drug (NSAID), such as Motrin (ibuprofen) or Aleve (naproxen), have a higher incidence of these complications.

HERE'S WHAT'S NEW • Researchers in Denmark have found that the selective serotonin reuptake inhibitors (SSRIs), the newest antidepressants, are associated with a significantly increased risk of gastrointestinal bleeding. These drugs, the best known of which are Prozac (fluoxetine) and Paxil (paroxetine), are widely used throughout the world. A study of 26,000 patients taking SSRIs found that these drugs caused stomach bleeding when taken alone and were especially risky when combined with either aspirin (5.2 times the incidence of bleeding) or an NSAID (12.2 times the risk). The researchers believe that some interaction between the antidepressant and the blood platelets accounts for this adverse effect.

> **THE BOTTOM LINE** • If you're taking an SSRI, report any stomach pain to your doctor and watch for evidence of bleeding from your intestinal tract—especially if you're older and also taking aspirin or an NSAID. Look for black stools, which indicate the presence of blood, and have them routinely checked by your doctor. (Note that iron supplements also can make stools black.) •

Are Antidepressants Safe during Pregnancy and Breastfeeding?

AS MANY AS 15 PERCENT of women of childbearing age are chronically depressed. Some even become suicidal. When such depression leads to alcoholism or illicit drug use during pregnancy or breastfeeding, it can have especially serious long-term consequences for a woman and her baby.

Normal brain function depends on an adequate supply of certain chemical "messengers," such as serotonin and norepinephrine, that transmit signals from one part of the brain to another. People with major depression have lower levels of these substances. The antidepressants, called selective serotonin reuptake inhibitors (SSRIs) can dramatically improve the mood and quality of life for depression sufferers by raising serotonin levels in the brain.

Is it safe for pregnant women and nursing mothers who need these drugs to take them?

HERE'S WHAT'S NEW

Even though SSRIs can be passed to the fetus via the bloodstream, research indicates that they do not increase risk of major birth defects or fetal death. However, to avoid withdrawal symptoms in newborns, some doctors recommend that these medications be tapered or discontinued 10 to 14 days before the patient's due date.

Doctors at the University of Bergen in Norway analyzed breast milk from 23 women who were taking an SSRI for depression while breastfeeding their babies. Blood samples from the mothers and children revealed that the drug was not present in breast milk or the babies' blood in appreciable amounts. The researchers conclude that these antidepressants are safe to take while nursing. In fact, they are especially useful in treating postpartum depression.

THE BOTTOM LINE

If you're seriously depressed while pregnant or breastfeeding, you may benefit from taking an SSRI at the lowest effective dose. But as with any medication, it's important for your doctor to monitor its use. You should also receive appropriate counseling and emotional support. Although some SSRIs, such as Prozac, may result in higher blood levels in the nursing infants than others (Paxil and Zoloft have the lowest concentrations in breast milk), none are high enough to harm the child.

DIABETES

· · · · · · · · · ·

You *Can* Prevent Diabetes

Monumental progress is being made in virtually every field of medicine. Vaccines, diagnostic equipment, surgical techniques, heart disease and cancer treatments . . . you name it, scientists are hard at work making life better. Advances in diabetes—ways to prevent it and better, easier ways to treat it—are also at the forefront of research.

Let's review the basics of this disease. There are two kinds of diabetes that appear to have totally different causes. Type 1 affects youngsters and is caused by the destruction of the cells in the pancreas that make insulin, a hormone that regulates glucose levels in the blood. The body's own immune system is responsible for this destruction, mistaking these cells for "enemy invaders." Until now, such autoimmune diseases have not been preventable. However, new research described in this chapter may change all that.

Type 2 (or adult-onset) diabetes accounts for 90 percent of cases. People with type 2 diabetes are able to make insulin, but it is unable to enter the body's cells and burn the glucose.

The end result in both types of diabetes is an elevated blood glucose level with all its consequences, the most important of which are generalized disease of blood vessels, and various neurologic abnormalities.

Type 2 diabetes can be prevented through weight loss, diet, and exercise. Diet is especially important and should include whole grains (as opposed to refined grains such as those in white bread) that increase the efficiency of insulin so that less is required to process glucose.

HERE'S WHAT'S NEW

Scientists have discovered an antibody that can stop the abnormal autoimmune response in type 1 diabetes from destroying the insulin-producing cells. This research is still in its early stages.

Scientists also are looking into the theory that type 1 diabetes is caused by an abnormal response of the body to some viral infection during childhood. If this is true, it may be possible to develop a vaccine that could prevent both the infection and the diabetes.

With regard to staving off type 2 diabetes, two drugs have been found useful. Glucophage (metformin), a prescription drug that limits the amount of glucose made by the liver, can help prevent diabetes in people who are obese, who have borderline blood glucose levels, and who have a family history of diabetes. However, it is not as effective as are weight loss, diet, and exercise.

Xenical (orlistat) is another drug useful in preventing type 2 diabetes in those especially vulnerable to the disease. It works by binding with the fat you've eaten after it reaches the stomach. As a result, the fat is not absorbed but passes out of the body in the stool along with the orlistat. Recent studies have shown that orlistat may play an important role in preventing heart disease, especially in diabetics, by reducing cholesterol levels and body weight.

THE BOTTOM LINE

If you're overweight and worried about developing diabetes because of a bad family history, or if you have a borderline blood glucose level, you can reduce your risk by getting lots of exercise, losing weight, and adding whole grains and nuts to your diet. Also, ask your doctor about taking metformin and orlistat, both of which also may prevent the onset of this disease. If you decide to use orlistat, take extra vitamins A, D, E, and K because these fat-soluble vitamins are excreted along with the dietary fat bound by orlistat.

A New Diabetes Home Test

THE SINGLE MOST IMPORTANT THING someone with diabetes can do to reduce the complications of their disease is to keep blood glucose levels as close to normal as possible. The easiest way to do so is to monitor blood sugar frequently using the fingerstick method. However, those results only tell you what's happening at that particular moment. Normal blood glucose at 2 P.M. does not necessarily indicate that it will remain normal the rest of the day—let alone the week.

To help patients control their blood glucose levels more efficiently over the long term, doctors use another blood test that measures glycolated hemoglobin (also referred to as hemoglobin A1c) about every 6 weeks. It reflects the average blood glucose level during the previous 6 to 12 weeks. Diabetics treated with insulin should have this test at least four times a year and more frequently if their blood glucose levels are difficult to control. Until now the glycolated hemoglobin test could only be done in the doctor's office.

HERE'S WHAT'S NEW

The FDA has approved Metrika A1c, the first over-the-counter test *you* can use to measure glycolated hemoglobin levels at home. It gives the result immediately.

THE BOTTOM LINE

I suggest that all diabetics take advantage of Metrika A1c. Medicare will pay for it as it does for most other routine diabetic supplies. Continue to use the fingerstick method to check your blood glucose level during the day, but test your hemoglobin A1c every 6 weeks for a better idea of how you're managing your diabetes over the long term.

No More Pins and Needles?

REGULAR MONITORING of the blood glucose level is the best way to keep diabetes under control and its ravages at bay. This means frequent finger-pricking to obtain a drop of blood for analysis. Most diabetics become resigned to it yet long for some device to do it noninvasively. Doctors also have been looking for alternatives to injectable insulin.

HERE'S WHAT'S NEW

The G2 Biographer from GlucoWatch can determine blood glucose levels noninvasively. Worn on the wrist, the device emits a low-level electric current that pulls glucose through the skin. It measures your sugar level for 13 hours, and sends an alarm whenever the reading is abnormal. (There's an equally interesting device already on the market in Europe that measures the blood glucose level using infrared rays directed at the skin. It is not yet available here.) The G2 can determine trends in your blood glucose and alert you to an impending significant drop, so you can adjust your insulin dosage and diet accordingly. Wearing the G2 at bedtime is especially useful to predict a dropping blood glucose level while you're asleep.

This device is not a substitute for the conventional skin prick that indicates your blood glucose level at any particular point in time. The G2 Biographer is meant to augment, rather than replace, conventional testing.

Considerable progress has also been made with regard to alternatives to injected insulin.

Insulin pills. Several pills and capsules now being tested can deliver insulin into the bloodstream within 20 minutes and lower blood glucose levels in patients with type 2 diabetes as effectively as injected insulin. They are not yet on the market, but probably will be in the near future.

Insulin spray. Insulin is delivered via inhalers similar to those used by asthmatics. The dose is absorbed by mucous membranes in the cheeks, tongue, and throat. The spray has been shown to work, and I predict its early approval, too.

Insulin patch. An electronic adhesive patch is first applied to the skin, where it painlessly vaporizes the cells on the surface, creating microscopic pores. Then a small insulin-coated patch is placed on the area, and the insulin is steadily absorbed through the openings for 12 hours. This is also an exciting prospect.

THE BOTTOM LINE

You can now buy a "watch" to wear on your wrist that gives you a good idea of how well your insulin dosage is correcting your blood glucose level. It is not as useful for assessing your glucose level at a specific time. You still need to prick your finger for that information.

You can look forward to taking your insulin by the oral, inhaled, or topical route instead of by injection before too long.

A Fishy Solution

DIABETES CAN LEAD to several life-threatening vascular complications—heart disease and stroke among them. The best way to avoid them is for diabetics to control their glucose levels and the other risk factors for vascular disease, such as high blood pressure, obesity, high cholesterol levels, physical inactivity, and tobacco use.

HERE'S WHAT'S NEW

Researchers from the Harvard School of Public Health and other Boston institutions studied more than 5,000 women with type 2 (adult-onset) diabetes enrolled in the Nurses Health Study to determine the impact of consuming the omega-3 fatty acids present in cold-water, oily fish on the cardiac complications of diabetes. None of the subjects had either heart disease or cancer at the onset of the study. During the next 16 years, diabetic women who ate this fish more than five times a week had a 64 percent reduction in heart attacks and overall mortality. Eating fish only one to three times a month led to a 30 percent lower risk of heart disease and death from any cause. Eating it once a week resulted in a 40 percent reduction.

THE BOTTOM LINE

In addition to controlling all risk factors for vascular disease, every diabetic should make a point of eating fish rich in the omega-3 fatty acids (mackerel, sardines, tuna, and salmon) at least once a week, and ideally, five or more times a week. (Pregnant women should not have mackerel, tuna, tilefish, swordfish, and shark because of their high mercury content—although canned light tuna is safe.) If fish is not your cup of tea, you can buy omega-3 fatty acids in capsule form. OmegaBrite, Solgar, and Twinlab are reliable brands.

The Promise of a Better Quality of Life

A DIABETIC'S LIFE is much better than it used to be. Home monitors for testing blood glucose levels have resulted in fewer attacks of low or high blood glucose levels, both of which frequently caused coma in the past. Years ago, when I was a resident in the emergency room, such cases were common. Sugar-lowering drugs as well as new forms of insulin have made blood glucose control smoother, with fewer peaks and valleys. But most important are the new discoveries on the horizon that promise to further reduce the complications of this disease and possibly even cure it.

HERE'S WHAT'S NEW

The most exciting news on the diabetes front is the result of work pioneered in Canada, where researchers in 1999 harvested insulin-producing pancreatic islet cells from fresh cadavers and transplanted them into patients with type 1 diabetes. This was done by injecting cells into the blood whence they traveled to the liver, where they continued to make insulin.

All of the first seven patients treated were able to discontinue insulin injections and enjoyed normal blood glucose levels.

Currently, researchers are evaluating 36 more patients treated with these islet cell injections. Results to date have varied depending on where the procedures were done. For example, 90 percent of those treated in Canada by the original researchers, as well as in a few American centers, no longer require insulin injections. However, in other locales, the success rate is only 3 out of 13. Hopefully, as doctors gain experience with this technique, the results will be more uniformly successful.

Although this concept is exciting and promising, there are some inherent problems. For example, harvesting the insulin-producing cells from a cadaver pancreas is difficult and time-consuming. These islet cells comprise only 3 to 4 percent of the millions of cells in each pancreas. They must be carefully "teased" from each fresh organ in a procedure that takes about 6 hours, and two cadavers usually are required to generate enough cells for one patient. Furthermore, after the cells are transferred, the recipient must take several anti-rejection drugs indefinitely, and these can have adverse effects.

In other news about breakthrough therapy for diabetes, scientists at the Centre for Regenerative Medicine at the University of Bath in the United Kingdom have developed a genetic-engineering process to transform human liver cells so that they make insulin. They are now looking to see whether these new cells can respond to fluctuating glucose levels in the blood. In the human body, when the blood glucose level is normal, the cells that make insulin reduce their production. As the blood glucose level rises, they produce more insulin. The question is whether these genetically engineered liver cells can also respond in this way. This entire project is early in its development, but it gives you some idea of the ingenious thoughts that occur to dedicated researchers.

There also may be a future in diabetes for stem-cell transplantation, transforming immature cells into insulin-producing tissues. This is probably the hottest area of research today for virtually every disease. Primitive cells that have not yet assumed an identity, derived either from embryos or normal bone marrow, are being introduced into damaged tissue in the hope they will grow to become—and ultimately replace—the cells that have been destroyed. To date, such stem cells have been injected into hearts whose muscle has been destroyed by heart attack as well as into brains that have been damaged by stroke or affected by diseases such as Parkinson's. There is considerable evidence that these stem cells can assume the identity of whatever tissue has been destroyed. Cells that make insulin will no doubt also be targeted.

THE BOTTOM LINE

If you have difficult-to-control type 1 diabetes that has begun to damage other organs such as the kidneys or the eyes, it's worth looking into islet cell transfer. The results have been encouraging, and it's only a matter of time until researchers refine the technique.

Genetic engineering and stem-cell transplantation are also on the horizon, and they look promising. My message to you now is that this research is ongoing and that a cure will one day be found.

WHAT THE DOCTOR ORDERED?

MULTIVITAMINS FOR DIABETICS WITH COLDS

Multivitamins are the epitome of the "quick fix" for which Americans are always looking. What harm, patients ask me, is there in popping one or two multivitamins every morning with breakfast? They aren't really drugs, are they? Multivitamins seduce so many of us mainly because they contain all the good things in the healthy foods that many of us never get around to eating—such as fruits and vegetables. As a result, at least 40 percent of Americans (who can afford them) take multivitamins.

Do multivitamins really do any good, or is it just wishful thinking? Several studies have attempted to answer that question. Unfortunately, the results are inconclusive because the goals of the studies are never quite clear. What do you look for when trying to decide whether a multivitamin is doing you any good? How you feel? That's pretty vague—and subject to many variables. And who can wait a lifetime to see whether the vitamins help people to live longer or better? So the studies' "end points"—that is, the things researchers measure to decide whether a given therapy is effective—are difficult to establish as far as multivitamin use is concerned.

Personally, I believe multivitamins are good (and actually necessary) for growing children, anyone who goes through life in and out of various crash diets, the elderly who live alone and whose nutrition may be compromised, and people who have documented nutritional deficiencies, such as those in developing countries.

HERE'S WHAT'S NEW • Doctors at the Carolinas Medical Center in Charlotte, North Carolina, undertook a research project that had a specific, well-defined goal: to determine whether an over-the-counter multivitamin had any effect on the immune systems (and therefore the resistance) of people with adult-onset, type 2 diabetes who were at least 45 years old. Such patients are generally more susceptible to viral and bacterial infections. Would the supplement protect them?

The answer in this small study was a resounding yes! The researchers found that only 17 percent of the diabetics who took a multivitamin developed a cold or other infection, while 93 percent of those receiving a placebo got sick. In a control group of subjects who were not diabetic, the supplement had no effect. In other words, it protected only the diabetics.

Why the difference in the responses of the diabetics and the control group? One possible explanation is that the elevated blood glucose level in diabetics interferes with the action of infection-fighting white blood cells, preventing them from killing bacteria and viruses as effectively. Another theory is that because diabetics urinate more frequently and copiously (in order for the body to eliminate excess glucose), they may excrete too much of certain substances that are thought to strengthen the immune system, including zinc and selenium. (People with diabetes have never been shown to be deficient in these chemicals.) The study findings are interesting regardless of how they're explained.

THE BOTTOM LINE • This small study will surely be repeated. In the meantime, if you have type 2 diabetes, there's no harm in taking a multivitamin once or twice a day. In fact, why not do so even if you have type 1 diabetes? Just make sure that the preparation contains some selenium and zinc, because they seem to be the major players. •

DIVERTICULAR
DISEASE

· · · · · · · · · ·

Conventional Wisdom Not So Wise

MANY WELL-MEANING DOCTORS continue to recommend erroneous treatments long after they should have been abandoned. The management of diverticular disease is a case in point.

Diverticulosis (outpouchings the size of large peas that develop in the colon) was first recognized in this country early in the 20th century, coincident with the introduction of processed food from which roughage had largely been removed. Diverticulosis is prevalent in other developed countries where most people eat predominantly low-fiber foods. By the same token, it's relatively uncommon in Africa and Asia where the diet is rich in fiber.

More than half the people over the age of 60 in this country have diverticulosis. Most of them are over 50, chronically constipated, and strain at stool. My patients tell me that they have been instructed to forgo foods such as raspberries, strawberries, nuts, and grapes, lest the seeds they contain get stuck in one of those pouches (diverticula) and inflame it. That advice is all wrong!

Diverticula usually don't cause symptoms, unless they become inflamed, infected, or leak into the abdominal cavity. However, they can thicken and can narrow the sigmoid (lower) portion of the colon, and cause chronic constipation with pelletlike stools, sometimes diarrhea, or intermittent spasm and pain in the left lower part of the belly. Whenever these pouches develop a painful infection, your diverticulosis becomes *diverticulitis*.

You're apt to learn that you have diverticulosis after undergoing an examination of the colon such as a colonoscopy, barium x-ray, or sigmoidoscopy. If your doctor's medical knowledge is out of date, that examination can change your life—for the worse—when you're advised to avoid healthy foods that you enjoy.

HERE'S WHAT'S NEW

The low-fiber, seedless diet for diverticulosis is passé. In fact, the very foods that are "prohibited" are exactly what most people with diverticulosis should eat! They eliminate the need to repeatedly force hard stool down, thus weakening areas of the bowel and causing them to bulge. The key to staving off diverticulosis or preventing it from becoming diverticulitis is to keep your bowels moving healthfully and regularly. Do that by slowly increasing the roughage in your diet until you reach about 35 grams of fiber daily, and drink eight 8-ounce glasses of water each day to wash it down.

Eat whole-bran cereal at breakfast and add more whole grains to your diet. Lots of berries, apples, and peaches, as well as vegetables such as broccoli, spinach, carrots, squash, and asparagus are also important. Beans and cabbage are controversial. Currently some doctors believe they're a good source of roughage, others say they simply cause gas and bloating.

THE BOTTOM LINE

Chances are you can keep your diverticulosis under control by eating more fiber or taking a stool-bulking agent such as psyllium (Metamucil, FiberCon, or others) or methylcellulose (Citrucel). Drink at least eight glasses of water a day and respond promptly when you "have to go."

ECZEMA

. . . .

Your Mom Could Have Prevented It

ECZEMA, OR ATOPIC DERMATITIS, is a chronic skin condition that affects about 10 percent of infants and children and 3 percent of adults in this country. You're more likely to have it if a close relative has it or suffers from hay fever, food allergies, or asthma. However, 20 percent of eczema patients have no such family history.

Teenagers and adults with eczema usually have dry, itchy easily irritated skin, with reddish-brown or gray, scaly, and thickened patches mostly on the hands and feet. In infants, the rash first appears on the face and scalp and often oozes and crusts. Once the baby begins crawling, exposed areas (such as the knees, elbows, ankles, wrists, and hands) are also affected.

Childhood eczema generally improves by age 25, but persists throughout life in 50 percent of cases. Itching is its most troublesome and common symptom in all age groups. (Incidentally, if you have a history of eczema, you should not have a smallpox vaccination—see page 346.)

Eczema is usually treated with topical medications—cortisone creams, ointments, lotions, and sometimes tars. Oral antihistamines may alleviate the itch. Antibiotics are necessary if the skin is infected. Dermatologists sometimes recommend treatment with ultraviolet light if the condition is severe. (Avoid oral steroids unless absolutely necessary. Their long-term use can result in a host of complications ranging from an impaired immune response to gastric bleeding and osteoporosis.)

A new class of medications called immunomodulators represents a major breakthrough in therapy for severe atopic dermatitis. Usually taken orally by transplant patients to help prevent organ rejection, these drugs can also clear up severe eczema when applied topically for long periods of time. The flagship drug in this category is Prograf (tacrolimus).

Patients with atopic dermatitis must learn how to take care of their skin. Food allergies play a role in some 30 percent of cases, so avoid foods that you know make your skin worse. Some substances in the environment—soaps, detergents, perfumes, cosmetics, even smoke—can also aggravate the rash either through contact or when inhaled. Neither skin testing nor allergy "shots" are usually of much help for eczema, so don't waste your time and money on them unless your dermatologist specifically recommends them.

HERE'S WHAT'S NEW

As noted on page 24, kids living in a compulsively clean environment during infancy are more likely to develop asthma and other allergic conditions. Eliminating every vestige of dust, mites, and other allergenic substances in the home prevents the body's immune system from "tooling" up. Unprovoked, our defenses slumber, then when attacked by the real thing, all hell breaks loose in the form of allergic reactions of one kind or another.

Assuming that eczema may also result from decreased bacterial exposure early in life, researchers decided to infect pregnant women with a "probiotic" (the opposite of an "antibiotic") called lactobacillus, a harmless infection that would activate their immune system and protect the fetus from atopic dermatitis. Doctors prescribe this innocuous organism for patients receiving long-term antibiotic therapy that kills good bacteria along with the harmful ones, leaving the field wide open for invasion by yeast and other organisms. Lactobacillus prevents this.

This study confirmed earlier findings that children born to mothers given lactobacillus just before delivery were 40 percent less likely to develop atopic dermatitis. This protection lasted at least until the child was 4 years old. (Note, however, that this beneficial effect protected the child only against atopic dermatitis, not asthma or other allergies.)

THE BOTTOM LINE

Atopic dermatitis is a lousy skin condition to have. The only good thing about it is the excuse it provides for you not getting the optional smallpox vaccine. Although there are many ways to treat this disorder, you're better off preventing it. If you're pregnant—and especially if you have a family history of allergy or atopic dermatitis—eat some yogurt (containing lactobacillus) or get your lactobacillus some other way (such as in a tablet) a few days before your delivery date. Studies suggest that this may reduce the risk of atopic dermatitis. Try it. You may like it.

ENDOMETRIOSIS

• • • • • • • • •

Surgical Relief for Runaway Menstruation

AFTER DECADES OF DEBATING the mystery of endometriosis, doctors finally understand a great deal more about this disease—a complex gynecological condition that affects an estimated 7 percent of
American females of reproductive age (more whites than blacks,
more Asians than whites).

Endometriosis is caused by tissue that normally lines the uterus
traveling locations where it has no business being—most commonly
the ovaries (in 75 percent of cases), the fallopian tubes (through
which the egg travels down from the ovaries to the uterus), or elsewhere in the pelvis—between the rectum and the vagina, in the
rectum itself, in the urinary bladder, in the appendix, and occasionally in the stomach. It has even been discovered in the gallbladder,
spleen, liver, and lungs. Imagine what it would be like if your heart

muscle migrated to your knee, or some lung tissue showed up in your elbow joint, or pieces of your brain traveled to your nose. You'd then have a beating knee, a breathing arm, and an intellectual schnoz.

Wherever this dislocated uterine tissue happens to end up, it sometimes behaves as if it were still in the uterus. That is, it menstruates! But unlike when it's in the uterus, blood has no way out of these other locations. So it forms scar tissue where it remains, and causes pain and irritation. Women with endometriosis suffer abdominal discomfort that interferes with sleep and results in persistent fatigue, they have mood swings, and intercourse is painful when endometrial tissue is present behind the uterus and the walls of the pelvis. Urination and bowel movements hurt, and these women may have premenstrual spotting, lower backache, and blood in the urine and stool. In some, endometriosis also interferes with the ability to have a baby if the misplaced tissue distorts the anatomy of the reproductive tract.

Much of the current focus in endometriosis research is on trying to determine what makes this tissue move. There is clearly a genetic component to it. If your sister or mother has endometriosis, there's a greater chance that you will too. However, some gynecologists think the disorder is due to an immune system abnormality that allows uterine cells to migrate and survive where they don't belong. There are other theories too. For example, it has been speculated that fluid containing these cells leaks out of the uterus and enters the bloodstream or the lymphatic system, spreading it throughout the body. According to another theory, during menstruation, in addition to flowing out of the uterus, some blood backs up into the fallopian tubes, onto the ovaries, and into the pelvis.

Other researchers blame the toxic substances in the environment, including dioxin (a chemical that may also produce cancer), environmental contaminants such as PCBs (polychlorinated biphenyls), and other "endocrine disrupters" that upset the normal hormonal balance. They point out that monkeys deliberately exposed to high concentrations of dioxin often develop endometriosis—and the greater the exposure, the more severe the disease. I believe these experimental data justify removing these pollutants from the environment.

Any disorder whose cause is not entirely clear and whose treatment is not always entirely satisfactory spawns misconceptions. For example, some of my patients have told me they suspect that intercourse during menstruation results in endometriosis (presumably by causing the flow of blood up into the fallopian tubes). There is no scientific basis for this belief. Another unlikely and unsubstantiated belief is that tampons and douching cause endometriosis.

Here's a piece of news that will surely startle you, as it did me. Endometriosis has been diagnosed in men! Yes, men. It appears that, very rarely, men with prostate cancer who are treated with high doses of estrogen may actually form endometrial tissue in their prostate glands. Of course, I'm not suggesting that men with abdominal cramps or gas pains should run out to see a gynecologist. But if you have recurrent, lingering, inexplicable symptoms and you have had high doses of estrogen—well, who knows?

HERE'S WHAT'S NEW

There is still no cure for endometriosis, but there are several treatments that can reduce pain, restore fertility, and shrink the amount of wandering tissue. Your doctor should suspect endometriosis if these symptoms are cyclical and coincide with menstruation. The most reliable way to diagnose endometriosis is by laparoscopy and biopsy, procedures that permit the doctor to view the pelvic and abdominal cavities, obtain tissue samples, and look at the tissue under the microscope. Vaginal ultrasound is another widely used diagnostic method. It is less expensive but not as reliable as laparoscopy.

Laparoscopy can be done at any time during the menstrual cycle. You are given an anesthetic, after which the doctor makes a small incision (about ¼ inch long), usually just below the navel. He or she then inserts a telescope-like thin, rigid tube about 12 inches long with a lens at the end attached to a light source. This permits a direct look at the uterus, ovaries, fallopian tubes, and other pelvic structures. If endometrial tissue is present, it is biopsied. Treatment should not be started until the tissue in question has been identified.

Although the most effective treatment for endometriosis is surgical removal of the offending tissue, if possible, surgery should be a last resort. Try medication first. The most effective drugs for pain relief are prostaglandin inhibitors, such as aspirin, and nonsteroidal anti-inflammatory drugs, such as Motrin (ibuprofen) and Aleve (naproxen). Tylenol (acetaminophen) may also help. The earlier you start taking such drugs after pain begins, the more effective they are. If the pain is very severe, you may need a prescription-strength painkiller.

Anything that blocks your periods will usually ease the symptoms of endometriosis. The most widely used agents that do so are the GnRH (gonadotropin-releasing hormones) agonists. They decrease the levels of luteinizing hormone and follicle-stimulating hormone, substances that stimulate the formation of estrogen. (Remember that estrogen makes the endometrial tissue grow.) GnRH, which takes about a month to start working, is marketed as a nasal spray called Synarel (nafarelin). It also can be injected into the muscle, as Lupron (leoprolide), or under the skin, as Zoladex (goserelin). The side effects of the GnRH drugs are what you would expect with a lack of estrogen: the kind of symptoms menopausal women have—hot flashes, insomnia, mild depression, breast tenderness, vaginal dryness, and reduced sex drive. Pregnant women should not take GnRH. The hormone progestin used to be popular but has been abandoned because the high doses required result in bloating, weight gain, depression, and irregular vaginal bleeding. It may also sometimes cause prolonged suppression of ovarian function even after it is stopped.

THE BOTTOM LINE

The benefits of medical therapy for endometriosis are usually transient. If it's possible to surgically remove or laser away enough endometrial tissue to make a difference, that's the way to go if medical management fails. The extent of the surgery will depend on the amount of wayward tissue and its location. If it's localized to a small area, it's no big deal. But sometimes, extensive surgery is required.

EYE PROBLEMS

· · · · · · · · ·

Keep Your Eyes on Fish

THE EYES ARE VULNERABLE to several unpleasant changes as we grow older. Among the most common are cataracts (easily removed by surgery), macular degeneration (commonly resulting in a wide array of vision loss often ending in blindness because treatment is not very successful), and dry eyes (uncomfortable, but manageable).

Macular degeneration is the leading cause of significant impaired vision in this country. About two million people, nearly all of whom are older than age 65, many with light-colored eyes, and mostly Caucasian can't see well because of it. About 165,000 new cases develop every year, around 16,000 of which result in blindness. The incidence is expected to triple by the year 2020, as the population ages.

The macula is a tiny area in the middle of the retina, situated in the back of the eye. When its cells degenerate, you have trouble seeing what is straight ahead of you and colors may appear dull. However, because the rest of the retina is not usually affected, you can still see out of the sides of the eyes, though not straight ahead. Now you know why some of your older friends prefer to sit beside the TV rather than in front of it.

Risk factors for macular degeneration are pollution, a high-fat diet sparse in fruits and vegetables, cigarette smoking, and a lifetime of excessive, unprotected exposure to bright sunlight. The best way for preventing it is to limit your exposure to these risks. There is some evidence that zinc supplements (80 milligrams a day) may also help prevent macular degeneration.

Dry eye syndrome affects over 10 million Americans and is basically a complication of aging. As we grow older, our bodies produce less oil—60 percent less at age 65 than at age 18. This decrease is more pronounced in women. As a result there is a decrease in the amount of oil in the tears that lubricate the eyes, causing tears to evaporate much more quickly. This leaves the cornea (the outermost layer of the eyes) abnormally dry and more easily scarred there by impairing vision.

Other factors besides age also contribute to dry eye syndrome. These include living in a hot, dry, windy climate or at high altitudes; continuous exposure to air-conditioning or cigarette smoke; and working long hours on a computer. Contact lenses also may be responsible because they can absorb tears and cause proteins to form on the surface of the lens. Low thyroid function, vitamin A deficiency, Parkinson's disease, and certain medications can all cause dryness too, as can low estrogen levels after menopause. The autoimmune disorder called Sjögren's syndrome is also characterized by dry eyes.

HERE'S WHAT'S NEW

Researchers at the National Eye Institute analyzed dietary data from more than 4,500 men and women ages 60 to 80. Those who regularly ate fish more than twice a week were half as likely to de-velop macular degeneration than those who ate no fish at all. Con-suming more than one portion of broiled or baked fish a week lowered the risk by one-third.

The researchers believe that a component of fish oil, the omega-3 fatty acid called docosahexaenoic acid (DHA), builds up in the eye near the light-sensing nerve cells of the macula and prevents their deterioration. Another report, this one from the Brigham and Women's Hospital in Boston, debunked a popularly held belief that beta-carotene supplements help prevent macular degeneration. More than 22,000 men followed for 12 years, half of whom were given such supplements, showed no reduction in the incidence of macular degeneration.

A diet rich in fish can also help dry eye syndrome. Harvard re-searchers analyzed data from more than 32,000 female health pro-fessionals in their Women's Health Study and found that those who consumed the most fish (and therefore the highest amount of omega-3 fatty acids) were least likely to have dry eye syndrome. This was es-pecially true for those women who ate the most fatty fish. Five or six 4-ounce servings of tuna a week lowered the risk by 66 percent!

THE BOTTOM LINE

This book is replete with examples of the many ways fish is good for you. The omega-3 fatty acids in fish lower blood pressure and cholesterol, and reduce the "clottability" of the blood. Add to all this the prevention of both a major cause of blindness in the United States as well as an unpleasant ocular condition, and you have a real winner. (Pregnant women should avoid mackerel, tuna, tilefish, swordfish, and shark because of their high mercury levels. Canned light tuna is safe.)

If you don't enjoy eating fish, you can buy omega-3 fatty acids in capsule form. But be sure to purchase a well-known brand, such as OmegaBrite, Solgar, Twinlab, and others. Unless properly made, the oil can become rancid.

Look for the Safest Glaucoma Treatment

GLAUCOMA IS A DISORDER in which the pressure of the fluid in the eyes is increased, eventually damaging the ocular nerve. It affects at least three million people in the United States—half of whom are unaware they have it. Glaucoma is the second leading cause of blindness in this country, accounting for 12 percent of all cases.

Tissues surrounding the lens of a healthy eye continuously produce a clear liquid called aqueous humor that keeps its interior moist. (This liquid has nothing to do with tears, which are made outside the eye and prevent its outer surface from drying.) Aqueous humor circulates in and out of the eye through the pupil, and is reabsorbed into the bloodstream through a meshwork of drainage canals around the outer edge of the iris (the colored part of the eye). Think of it as a sink with the faucet turned on. The tissues that produce the fluid are the faucets and the drainage canals of the eye (like the drain pipes connected to the sink), preventing it from overflowing. They must remain open and unobstructed.

The internal pressure in the eye depends on how much fluid it contains and whether it can pass freely in and out. As we grow older, the drainage canals begin to function less effectively. They also angle and bend, interfering with flow through them. As a result, fluid backs up and stagnates within the eye, raising its pressure. This condition, called *primary open-angle glaucoma*, accounts for at least 60 percent of glaucoma seen in the elderly. It is an insidious process that rarely causes any symptoms until the optic nerve has been damaged and vision lost. Once that happens, sight cannot be restored, so prevention and early treatment are key. *Increased pressure in the eye results in glaucoma only if has been undetected and left untreated for any length of time.*

The more serious but much less common form of glaucoma is *acute angle-closure glaucoma*. Instead of a slow, progressive buildup of fluid pressure within the eye, the canals become obstructed suddenly. This results in a variety of acute symptoms, including loss of vision, pain in the eyes, headache, nausea and vomiting, and rainbow halos when you look at lights. *This is a medical emergency.* Unless it is treated quickly, blindness can occur within hours.

Fortunately, glaucoma is easy to diagnose and treat. All you need to do is see an ophthalmologist regularly after age 35. If you're found to have elevated intraocular pressure, it can be normalized with several kinds of eyedrops. The most widely used are the beta-blockers, an example of which is Timoptic (timolol). They lower eye pressure by decreasing production of aqueous humor.

Beta-blockers also are taken by mouth and by injection to treat heart failure, lower high blood pressure, and manage certain cardiac rhythm disorders. They're called beta-blockers because they block the production of adrenaline-like substances that help control heart rate and prevent the bronchial tubes from going into spasm. Someone taking a beta-blocker is likely to have a slower heart rate and, if he or she has some underlying pulmonary problem, can develop wheezing and respiratory difficulties. Beta-blockers also can interact adversely with other cardiac drugs such as calcium channel blockers and digitalis.

What does this have to do with treating glaucoma? Whenever a medication is introduced into the eye, some of it is absorbed through the tear ducts and enters the body's circulation. When prescribing a beta-blocker for heart patients, doctors first make sure that the drug is safe for them. However, a patient's vulnerability to the adverse effects of beta-blockers is not always taken into account when the drug is prescribed as an eyedrop. The problem is further compounded by the fact that many people have respiratory problems of which they are unaware or that are not obvious, especially to an eye doctor. In such cases, beta-blocker eyedrops can have serious consequences similar to those caused when administered orally.

HERE'S WHAT'S NEW

Researchers at the Institute of Ophthalmology in London compared the findings in 2,600 glaucoma patients being treated with beta-blocker eyedrops with 9,000 people who had normal eye pressure. Those taking the drops, many of whom had no known history of lung problems, had a greater incidence (1 in every 55) of respiratory symptoms that required medical attention than those who did not receive a beta-blocker.

THE BOTTOM LINE

These observations, which affect hundreds of thousands of people being treated for glaucoma, are significant. Although beta-blockers are among the most widely used drops to lower intraocular pressure, some people clearly should not be taking them.

Before you start one of these drugs, I strongly suggest that you have a spirometry (breathing) test. Most eye specialists don't routinely perform it, so you'll have to ask your general practitioner or internist to arrange it. A normal spirometry reading is fairly good evidence that it's safe for you to take beta-blocker eyedrops—as far as your lungs are concerned. But don't forget your heart. Ask your internist if any of your other medications can interact with a beta-blocker. Also, if you've been told you have a slow heart rate, make sure it's monitored after you start the beta-blocker. Remember too that lung problems can develop at any time as you get older, so it's a good idea to have your lung function and your pulse rate checked periodically while you're taking the drug.

If for some reason you aren't a good candidate for beta-blocker therapy for your glaucoma (because you have lung disease or your heart rate is too slow), other treatment options are available. These include carbonic anhydrase inhibitors, prostaglandin analogs, alpha-2 agonists, and cholinergic drugs. Discuss them with your eye doctor.

If the increased pressure within the eye cannot be reduced with medication, several surgical laser procedures are available.

FIBROMYALGIA

· · · · · · · · ·

Leave No Stone Unturned

Sometimes the biggest breakthrough in a disease is getting the medical community to believe it even exists! Such has been the case with fibromyalgia, or fibromyalgia syndrome (FMS)—an ailment so elusive and mysterious that until recently, those unfortunate enough to suffer from it were often stigmatized as neurotics.

We now know that fibromyalgia affects more than six million Americans, more than 75 percent of whom are women, mostly in their forties or fifties. They suffer a host of symptoms that would make the most macho men cry: deep, severe aching or burning muscular pain, persistent fatigue, poor sleeping patterns, depression, and often a "nervous stomach" associated with bouts of diarrhea or constipation.

Despite all this, they don't *look* sick! These people have no fever, they eat well, and they maintain their weight. Their joints are not arthritic despite the pain; there is no evidence of any connective-tissue disease such as lupus despite the wide array of symptoms; their thyroid function is normal and does not account for their fatigue; and every conceivable test comes back normal. In short, fibromyalgia leaves no objective evidence of its presence. Patients go from doctor to doctor, desperately looking for an explanation, trying to understand why they feel so lousy. After a thorough and careful workup reveals no abnormalities, most of them are told, "There's nothing wrong with you" or "It's all in your head."

We now know better. If you've had most of the following symptoms for at least 3 months, you probably have FMS:

- Deep, aching pain in various parts of the body: the neck, between the shoulder blades, the shoulders themselves, the hips, the knees. This is the sine qua non of fibromyalgia. *You must have pain for this diagnosis to be appropriate*
- Inordinate fatigue for no apparent reason, worse in the morning than later in the day
- Trouble falling asleep, and then waking frequently during the night
- Joint pain
- Frequent headaches
- Urinary frequency
- Restless legs or leg cramps (or both)
- Anxiety or depression
- Painful menstrual periods (premenstrual syndrome)
- Diarrhea and constipation
- Sensitivity to heat, cold, and changes in humidity
- Chronic sore throat

- Difficulty concentrating and impaired memory

- Mottled skin

- Sensitivity to bright light, odors, and loud sounds

A key diagnostic finding shared by all fibromyalgia patients is their "trigger points": discrete, painful little knots in the muscles. These trigger points can be located in any muscle of the body—in the neck (where they may be mistaken for a tension headache), on the hips or buttocks, or around the knees and elbows. They are generally symmetrical—that is, when present on one side of the body, they have a similar distribution on the other.

Although multiple symptoms of FMS are typical, do not accept this diagnosis until other possible and treatable causes have been ruled out. These include thyroid dysfunction (over- or underactive), several neurological disorders, connective-tissue diseases such as scleroderma, certain forms of arthritis, and even cancer.

Although if you have FMS, chances are that one of your blood relatives does too, as of now, no specific FMS gene has been identified. There also seems to be some relationship between fibromyalgia and acute stress.

Currently, there are several different theories to explain FMS, all of which have their passionate advocates but none of which are universally accepted. Blood tests may reveal a deficiency of tryptophan, the precursor of serotonin (a chemical in the brain that transmits nerve messages, inhibits pain perception, and induces deep sleep). The problem is that serotonin levels are also low among those suffering from depression without FMS. Some researchers believe that FMS is caused by a viral or other infection, but the responsible agent has not been identified. Others suspect that FMS is a disorder of the immune system, but again they have not been able to prove it.

There is no cure for FMS. Its symptoms wax and wane but almost never clear up. Certain medications can improve the quality of life for some suffering from FMS. The most effective agents in the management of FMS are those that raise the level of serotonin. The most widely used is the tricyclic antidepressant Elavil (amitriptyline), in a dose of 25 to 75 milligrams taken at bedtime. Also useful are selective serotonin reuptake inhibitors (SSRIs), the prototype of which is Prozac (fluoxetine). They work by raising the serotonin levels in the brain and prolonging stage 4 sleep, thus promoting deep slumber. Tofranil (imipramine) and Desyrel (trazodone) also help. Unfortunately, painkillers such as aspirin or nonsteroidal anti-inflammatories are not really effective. Avoid the use of narcotics and barbiturate sleeping pills that can lead to habituation or addiction.

You may obtain temporary relief by having your trigger points injected with a local anesthetic such as lidocaine and then stretching the involved muscle. However, there are too many of these trigger points for this technique to be of much practical help over the long term.

Eat a well-balanced diet. Cut back on sugar, too much of which can reduce your energy level. Avoid acid-forming foods, red meat, carbonated drinks, and caffeine. On theoretical grounds you should keep away from any food to which you are allergic. Also make sure you consume enough protein, as this nutrient is necessary for tissue repair.

HERE'S WHAT'S NEW

Anyone suffering from a chronic and incurable disorder such as FMS is a target for unscrupulous promoters who can make any product sound reasonable. The Internet is full of such ineffective remedies, most of which are supplements and herbs. On the positive side, research indicates that essential fatty acid supplements such as gamma linolenic acid (GLA) may improve symptoms in some patients.

More questionable is the use of guaifenesin for the treatment of FMS. There have been several reports and at least two books written about it. You may know guaifenesin as Robitussin, a popular cold remedy that helps loosen mucus in the respiratory system. It is said to work in FMS by reducing calcium phosphate deposits in muscles and other tissues and acting on the kidneys so that they excrete them. I have not read a properly documented scientific study to substantiate this theory. What's more, I'm not aware of any sophisticated diagnostic techniques that detect the presence of such deposits. A double-blind study on 23 patients revealed that guaifenesin did not increase phosphate excretion and was no more effective than a placebo.

Several studies highlight the importance of exercise and relaxation for alleviating the symptoms of FMS. Regular exercise is extremely important, not only for pain relief but also because it promotes stage 4 sleep, the deepest level that the body needs to repair damaged and aging tissue, produce antibodies, and make enough hormones, neurotransmitters, and immune system chemicals. So do some form of exercise, such as walking or cycling, every day. Gentle exercise in water is preferable to jogging or weight lifting. Most patients who perform such exercises along with relaxation therapy (described below) do feel better. But don't do too much too soon. I usually refer patients with FMS to specially trained physiatrists (medical doctors who specialize in physiotherapy) for advice on an appropriate exercise regimen.

Some patients are helped by transcutaneous electrical nerve stimulation (TENS), in which electrodes are applied to the body to stimulate nerves and relieve pain. Moist heat from hot packs, warm baths, heating pads, or whirlpool baths at a physiotherapy clinic also relieve pain. Gentle massage is beneficial too. All of these therapies work better if you also try to reduce your stress level. Meditational yoga, biofeedback, and various relaxation exercises, the best known of which is Herbert Benson's Relaxation Response, described in his books, are good too, as is acupuncture (or acupressure).

THE BOTTOM LINE

However you choose to treat your fibromyalgia, remember that your symptoms are not all in your head. There's no reason to be ashamed of your illness. Seek active medical care even though the cause of your disease remains unknown and there is no specific cure for it. Do not allow yourself to be deprived of any intervention that can help you. You are not a hypochondriac; you are not a neurotic. You are entitled to receive whatever (little) modern medicine can do for you. Get a thorough evaluation of your symptoms to exclude some other disease that might possibly account for your misery; see a physiatrist for help with an exercise program; take advantage of the various therapeutic agents that can ease your suffering. But be careful about seeing a "fibromyalgia specialist." There's no such thing. Find a doctor who believes you, who agrees that fibromyalgia is a real disorder, and who will leave no stone unturned to help you.

GALLBLADDER
DISEASE

· · · · · · · · ·

Leave Well Enough Alone

TWENTY MILLION AMERICANS (about 9 percent of the population) have some problem with their gallbladders—stones, infection, or irritation. Each year about 500,000 of them have it removed. That number would be even higher were it not for some new light shed on this old disease.

Until fairly recently, we used to recommend removing the gallbladder whenever it contained stones (usually composed of cholesterol). We assumed they'd inevitably act up sometime in the future and cause pain, fever, chills, nausea, vomiting, and frequently jaundice and pancreatitis. Doctors generally felt that a patient was a better operative risk at the time of diagnosis than some time in the future. That suggestion would make sense if gallstones did, in fact, always act up. We now know that, each year, only 2 percent of them actually do so. The current thinking is that it's better to leave "silent" gallbladder disease alone unless symptoms keep recurring. There are measures to prevent the problem from requiring surgery—and to reduce the likelihood of stones forming in the first place.

If any of the following risk factors apply to you, start taking steps to reduce your chance of developing gallbladder disease:

- Men and women who weigh too much are three to seven times more likely to form gallstones, probably because their gallbladders are sluggish and their bile contains more cholesterol.

- By the time they reach 80, 10 percent of men and more than 20 percent of women have gallstones.

- Females between the ages of 20 and 60 are at least twice as vulnerable as men are.

- Pregnancy is associated with increased gallstone formation due to some mechanism that is not fully understood.

- Diabetics with high triglyceride levels are more vulnerable to gallstones.

- Birth control pills and estrogen replacement therapy raise the risk of gallstones because estrogen increases the blood cholesterol level and decreases contractility of the gallbladder. That means the organ doesn't "squeeze" as vigorously, so the bile it contains (and its cholesterol) becomes sluggish and forms stones.

- Certain medications that lower cholesterol, such as Abitrate (clofibrate), increase its concentration in the bile, raising the risk of gallstones in both men and women. (This does not apply to the cholesterol-lowering "statin" drugs.)

• Most Native American men have gallstones by the time they're 60; 70 percent of female Pima Indians from Arizona develop gallstones by age 30; and Mexican-Americans of any age and both genders are also vulnerable to stone formation because their bile is very rich in cholesterol.

• The liver secretes extra cholesterol and tends to form cholesterol stones in people who have been following a very low calorie diet (less than 800 calories per day for 12 to 16 weeks). Stones may also form after gastric bypass surgery. In one study, 38 percent of those who underwent such surgery developed gallstones within a few months. Women who lose between 19 and 22 pounds over a 2-year period are 44 percent more likely to develop gallstones too.

If you're vulnerable, avoid fat in your diet. Every time fat globules (in butter, bacon, cream, and marbled steak, for example) reach the small intestine, they send signals calling for more bile. That requires the gallbladder to contract, increasing the risk of dislodging a stone that already happens to be there. Even in the absence of stones, a fatty meal (or spicy food) will usually result in gas, bloating, and indigestion if your gallbladder isn't functioning normally.

Suspect gallstones if you develop chronic indigestion, nausea, bloating, and lots and lots of burping after a fatty meal. Many people go through life with these symptoms, in the mistaken belief that they were born that way.

If you have gallstones and they act up, these medications will relieve your symptoms:

- Antispasmodics such as Bentyl (dicyclomine) relax the muscles of the gastrointestinal tract. The usual dose is anywhere from 10 to 40 milligrams taken orally three or four times a day. This is a prescription drug and your doctor will know whether it is safe for you to take it. Robinul (glycopyrrolate)—one tablet three times a day—acts in much the same way. Avoid Bentyl if you have glaucoma, active angina, ulcerative colitis, or a big hiatus hernia with lots of acid reflux.

- For nausea, try Compazine (prochlorperazine) in a dose of 5 to 10 milligrams every 4 hours, as needed. Be careful with it if you have heart disease or narrow angle glaucoma. Phenergan (promethazine) is also effective in doses of 12.5 to 25 milligrams. Avoid it if you have active heart disease, asthma, or impaired liver function. You'll need prescriptions for both these medications.

- There are various analgesics for pain relief, ranging all the way from Tylenol (acetaminophen) and aspirin to narcotics such as Demerol (meperidine).

HERE'S WHAT'S NEW

If you're having frequent attacks, your best option is laparoscopic surgery. (Ask for a second opinion if you're offered the old, more invasive surgical procedure.) In laparoscopic surgery, the surgeon makes four incisions in the abdomen, each only about ½ inch long. A tiny video camera is then introduced into one of the incisions. It sends back a magnified image of what it sees within the abdomen. The surgeon then inserts various instruments through the other incisions, using them to separate the gallbladder from the liver and all ducts in the area, and then removing it. In about 5 percent of cases, the camera reveals scarring or infection that make the invasive operation necessary.

There are other options for dealing with symptomatic gallstones. A few medical centers are using lithotripsy to shatter single stones that are less than an inch in size. This procedure is fairly new in the United States, but it has been around for about 15 years in Austria, where it was developed. I don't recommend it. The shocks do fragment the stones, but at a high price. Smaller pieces can enter the ducts, where they can cause more trouble than did the one large stone, at least over the short term. Ten to 40 percent of stones recur after lithotripsy.

Ursodiol (ursodeoxycholic acid) is another treatment. It comes in a pill form and dissolves the stones. Again, it's not as effective as we initially hoped it would be. And even if it does dissolve the stones, there's no guarantee that new ones won't form in the future. In fact, they do so in about half the patients treated.

Here's a new finding that is potentially very important: Scientists have determined that a single large stone in your gallbladder may predispose you to cancer of that organ. I tell my patients about this possibility, and together we decide what to do. I usually recommend removal of the gallbladder in such cases even if there are no symptoms and despite the fact that the risk of cancer is low.

THE BOTTOM LINE

Gallstones occur more frequently as one gets older—and more commonly in women (especially those taking estrogen), Native Americans, Mexican-Americans, and people who yo-yo their weight with crash starvation diets. Gallstones do not usually cause symptoms. Fever, jaundice, and right-side abdominal pain are the hallmarks of an acute attack.

If your gallstones don't bother you, let them be. If attacks recur, have your gallbladder removed via laparoscopy, a minimally invasive technique. The older, major operation is now done only when laparoscopy is not possible due to scarring or infection in and around the gallbladder.

There are nonsurgical ways to treat gallstones, but their success is unpredictable and they are not as effective as surgery.

The key fact to remember is that the mere presence of gallstones does not mean that you need an operation. If such stones are found incidentally during a routine x-ray of the abdomen and you're advised to have surgery, get a second opinion.

GASTROESOPHAGEAL REFLUX DISEASE (GERD)

· · · · · · · · ·

Relief at Last

MILLIONS OF AMERICANS—as many as 20 percent of the population—suffer from the reflux of stomach acid into the food pipe. When the muscle in your lower esophagus is weak and doesn't close properly, acid, food, and liquid spill up from the stomach and into the food pipe. Doctors call it gastroesophageal reflux disease (GERD). Signs and symptoms include heartburn, choking, chest pain, and burping, all of which are usually worse when you lie down after a meal. You can control these symptoms with antacids, medications that reduce stomach acid production, and various maneuvers such as

147

elevating the head of your bed to reduce the amount of acid reflux when you lie down.

I'm amazed at how often a problem in one system of the body can affect other seemingly unrelated functions. For example, someone with premature heart disease may have a horizontal crease in each ear lobe. Or someone with jaundice due to liver disease or gallbladder duct obstruction may itch all over. Here are some other examples involving GERD.

Researchers found that among a group of 330 patients with obstructive sleep apnea—a condition of disturbed sleep patterns during which breathing stops for as long as 10 seconds, is followed by a gasp, and then resumes once more—62 percent of them also had GERD.

Patients with obstructive sleep apnea usually are treated with continuous positive airway pressure (CPAP). They are fitted with a mask attached to a machine that delivers pressurized air (not oxygen) through the nostrils. This keeps the airways open and prevents the breathing interruptions.

HERE'S WHAT'S NEW

Recent studies have shown that almost half the patients with sleep apnea who also have GERD experience improvement in their gastric reflux symptoms when their sleep problem is treated with CPAP. That shouldn't come as a surprise. By increasing pressure in the chest, CPAP prevents acid from backing up into the esophagus.

Researchers have recently developed a special liquid polymer (a chemical found in myriad products ranging from hair spray to plastic) that can be injected into the lower esophagus. It strengthens the muscle fibers so they stay shut and prevent reflux.

The manufacturers of this drug (marketed under the brand name Enteryx) reported to the FDA that it effectively reduces symptoms of GERD, at least over the short term. Patients treated with it required fewer antacids and similar drugs. One year after receiving the injection, two-thirds of patients were able to get along without any medication. Enteryx apparently has no major adverse effects (at least in the first year), though some patients did complain of irritation of the esophagus for months after the injection. The FDA has approved Enteryx for use in the United States.

And the simplest news yet: Chewing gum can also provide temporary relief of GERD symptoms. According to researchers at Kings College in London, it does so first by stimulating swallowing that in turn helps clear acid from the food pipe. Second, and perhaps more important, it also increases secretion of saliva. The alkaline saliva neutralizes some of the excess acid in the upper gastrointestinal tract.

THE BOTTOM LINE

If you have both GERD and sleep apnea, and haven't gotten enough relief of your indigestion symptoms from conventional therapy, try CPAP at night.

When symptoms are severe and persistent, ask your doctor about Enteryx. When it's injected into the lower esophageal muscle, it may strengthen the muscle sufficiently to reduce the upward leak of acid.

In addition to everything else you do for your GERD, chew some gum, even though Medicare probably won't reimburse you for it.

GOUT

· · · · · · · · ·

An Equal Opportunity Offender

Gout has often been referred to as "the disease of kings and the king of diseases." That's because gout attacks—which are a "royal" pain!—usually result from bingeing on the kind of rich food and alcoholic drink that would befit a king.

Here's how a typical incident plays out: You're a man in your fifties, you're a little overweight, and you love to eat. One evening, you enjoy an exceptionally gratifying meal—a 3-pound lobster washed down with a couple of beers and topped off with a delicious banana split. Drowsy with satiated delight, you hit the sack. Before you can begin to dream, you awake with a pain in your right big toe. It's so excruciating you can't bear to have the bedsheet touch it. Suddenly, now fully awake, you remember your father—and his attacks of gout. Like father, like son!

Gout is a common form of arthritis caused by excess uric acid, a small amount of which is normally present in the bloodstream. It comes from purine, the waste by-product of normal cell death that occurs constantly in the body. It's also present in certain foods. Because our kidneys are constantly excreting the uric acid that we eat or that the body makes, we are normally able to maintain a level in the blood of between 2 and 7 milligrams per cubic centimeter. That number increases when the body makes more uric acid than the kidneys can eliminate (usually because they're diseased) or we eat far too many purine-containing foods, such as meat (veal, venison, and bacon), turkey, animal organs, seafood, nuts, and dried legumes.

Whatever the origin, high uric acid levels in the blood cause needlelike crystals of uric acid to form in various joints, most commonly the big toe but also in the foot, ankle, heel, knee, elbow, wrist, or finger. The immune system tries to get rid of these crystals by unleashing a barrage of defense mechanisms. Swarms of white blood cells attack and engulf them, and as they do so, they release enzymes that cause inflammation. It's this vigorous counterattack and these enzymes—not the crystals themselves—that cause the pain. The gout attack usually peaks within 1 to 2 days and, if left alone, it gradually subsides within 7 to 10 days after the immune system has abandoned its fruitless countermeasures.

HERE'S WHAT'S NEW

Despite the image of gluttony, booze, and obesity, we now know that gout usually is not caused by lifestyle; it's in the genes. But if you have a genetic predisposition, your behavior can bring on an attack. In the United States, the incidence of gout is 2.7 in every 1,000 adults; in England, that figure is 19.3 per 1,000. Gout is even more common among the Maoris of New Zealand and among Pacific Islanders, 10 percent (or 100 in 1,000) of whose men suffer from it.

Gout is much more common in men over the age of 45, with a male-to-female ratio of 9 to 1. It rarely occurs in premenopausal women.

Even though excess uric acid in the blood is the problem, you can have an attack of gout even if your uric acid level is normal. So don't dismiss a gout diagnosis just because your uric acid level isn't elevated. By the same token, if you have joint pains that don't really look like gout but are diagnosed as such because your uric acid level is high, consult an arthritis specialist (rheumatologist). To firmly establish the diagnosis, a rheumatologist may withdraw some fluid from the affected joint and look for the presence of the uric acid crystals under the microscope.

Gout attacks usually recur if the disease is not managed properly (only 5 to 10 percent of patients have only one attack), and they eventually damage the joints and the kidneys. Uric acid crystals don't settle only in the joints; they can also accumulate on tendons and ear cartilage, where they form lumps or nodules called *tophi*. Crystals can also coalesce to form uric acid stones in the kidneys.

Modern medications can usually prevent attacks of gout. The most effective therapy these days is the nonsteroidal anti-inflammatory drugs (NSAIDs), such as Motrin (ibuprofen) and Aleve (naproxen). The over-the-counter strength usually isn't enough, so you'll have to ask your doctor for a prescription for a more potent dose. The longer you wait to begin treatment, the less effective it is, so get medical help right away. In addition to taking medication, drink five or six glasses of water, rest, and elevate the affected limb. Continue the NSAID until the pain subsides, then go on to a different group of drugs that prevents recurrent attacks.

There is a drug you should take on an ongoing basis to keep the uric acid within normal limits and reduce the likelihood of acute gout. (Remember that repeated episodes, even if you're stoic and able to withstand the pain, ultimately can damage your joints and your kidneys.) Zyloprim (allopurinol) is a long-term medication that prevents the purines in your food from converting to uric acid. It is effective and very well-tolerated. Another medication, Benemid (probenecid), reduces uric acid levels by increasing the acid's excretion by the kidneys. If your doctor prescribes Benemid, stop taking aspirin, because it interferes with the drug.

Because these drugs may initially increase the risk of an attack, it's a good idea to also take one or two colchicine tablets a day along with them for the first few weeks after starting any of them. Colchicine is extracted from the autumn crocus and, for many years, was all we had to treat gout. It's not used routinely anymore for acute attacks because it causes a host of unpleasant side effects. However, in small doses colchicine is usually well-tolerated.

While in the midst of an acute attack, do not take any agent that lowers uric acid. Avoid aspirin, diuretics (water pills), alcohol, Sinemet (levodopa-carbidopa) for the treatment of Parkinson's disease, nicotinic acid (to lower cholesterol), cyclosporine (an anti-rejection drug marketed as Neoral), the anti-tuberculosis medications pyrazinamide (sold as a generic drug) and ethambutol (Myambutol). They all may worsen symptoms by interfering with uric acid excretion.

If you choose not to take any maintenance or preventive therapy, avoid purine-rich foods and reduce or eliminate alcohol. But you'd better keep your fingers crossed. This strategy works only in a lucky 10 percent of patients—60 percent have a recurrence within a year, and almost 80 percent get another attack within 2 years unless they're on a drug such as Zyloprim (allopurinol).

THE BOTTOM LINE

If you suddenly have an acutely painful joint that has all the characteristics of gout, see your doctor as soon as possible, because treatment is most effective when started early. A normal uric acid level does not rule out the diagnosis, and a high one doesn't always confirm it. If you're having symptoms suggestive of gout but your uric acid level is normal, see an arthritis specialist or orthopedist. You may need to have the fluid in the affected joint removed and analyzed for the presence of the characteristic needlelike uric acid crystals.

Another condition, called pseudogout, caused by deposits of calcium crystal (not uric acid crystal) in the joints closely mimics gout. It's important to distinguish between the two because, despite their striking similarity, their long-term management is different. Withdrawing fluid from the joint and examining the crystals establishes the proper diagnosis.

HAIR LOSS

• • • • • • • • •

To Have or Not to Have

Two of every three men develop a receding hairline by the time they're 50, and—lest you think hair loss is a bane only to men—more than a third of American women also experience significant hair loss.

"Natural" pattern, or hereditary baldness (androgenic alopecia), used to be considered incurable, but there are now several ways to deal with it. What's more, some non-hereditary, hair-losing conditions may be reversible.

HERE'S WHAT'S NEW

The most recent medical treatment for baldness is Propecia (finasteride). Unlike an earlier drug Rogaine (minoxidil), Propecia works only in men. It is a weaker strength of Proscar, the 5-milligram dose of which is prescribed to help shrink an enlarged prostate and reduce the frequency of night visits to the john. The FDA approved finasteride for the treatment of hair loss in men at the end of 1997. The dose is a daily 1-milligram tablet. In one new report, two years of therapy with Propecia resulted in longer and thicker hair in 66 percent of men, and further hair loss was arrested in five of every six of them. You'll also be happy to note, it doesn't increase hair growth anywhere but on your head.

Propecia acts by blocking an enzyme called 5-alpha-reductase that converts the male hormone testosterone to dihydrotestosterone (DHT), which causes baldness. Propecia reduces the amount of DHT in your body, usually without decreasing masculinity. However, some men do occasionally become impotent or lose some of their sexual desire after using it.

Propecia is available only by prescription and costs about twice as much as Rogaine (about $50 per month as compared to $20 or less). Remember that it is not meant for women or children. It should never be taken or even handled by any female who is either pregnant or potentially so, since it can cause abnormalities of the genital tract in the fetus.

Some men in this country have recently started taking saw palmetto, an herb used for treating symptoms of prostatic enlargement, to try to block the 5-alpha-reductase enzyme, much as does Propecia. However, evidence that it prevents hair loss is still sparse.

Rogaine is still available—and you can now buy it over-the-counter. It can be more effective in women than in men. However, about 10 to 14 percent of males who use it do obtain visible regrowth; others stop losing their hair, or do so more slowly. In some cases, it only maintains the status quo—things just don't get worse.

As a last resort, if other methods of preventing baldness don't work, consider hair transplantation. This usually involves moving hair from the back of the scalp to the bald spot. There are several different kinds of procedures such as scalp reduction and flap surgery, depending on the hair geography of your scalp, and they're usually done by a dermatologist. I have seen the most natural results transplanting hair with "micro grafts" using up to 4 hairs per graft. But be sure to check the cost before you decide to go this route. It's expensive and not usually covered by insurance.

What if your hair loss isn't hereditary? Hair loss is much less common in China, Italy, and Japan than it is in America. Although that's partly due to genetic differences, diet also plays a part. Our American eating habits may be showing up on our heads as well as our waistlines. Hairier populations generally eat more leafy green vegetables, fish, unsaturated fats, and antioxidants such as vitamins C and E than we do—foods that nourish hair and promote its growth.

Thyroid malfunction is another common culprit in hair loss. Thyroid trouble is the first thing to look for when your basin and pillow are covered with hair. Ask for a simple blood test of thyroid function. If it's too low or too high, replacing the missing hormone or cutting down its overproduction returns your body metabolism to normal and your hair may stop falling out. Many other diseases and medications can cause temporary hair loss as well (tell your doctor about any unusual hair loss). In most cases, hair can grow back.

THE BOTTOM LINE

Hair loss is essentially a cosmetic problem—no one ever died from baldness or thinning hair—but it can also reflect an underlying disorder. That's why you should have a complete physical examination if you have unexplained hair loss.

For plain old hereditary baldness, try the newest drugs available (such as Propecia), so long as they're deemed safe in your particular case. Otherwise, if you've done all you can and you simply don't like the way you look, consider hair transplantation, but don't expect your insurance company to reimburse you for it.

HEART DISEASE

· · · · · · · · ·

New Treatments for Weak Hearts

THE MAIN FUNCTION OF THE HEART is to pump oxygen-rich blood to every part of the body—around the clock, every day of the year, for as long as you live. However, several conditions can weaken the force with which it does so, including a previous heart attack; long-standing untreated high blood pressure (against which the heart has been pumping to get its blood into the arteries); damage to one or more of the four heart valves; a disease of the heart muscle itself (cardiomyopathy); infections, mostly viral; and other conditions that involve and injure the heart muscle.

When cardiac function has been compromised for any reason, the heart tries to maintain its ability to expel the necessary amounts of blood by enlarging and becoming thicker. When it can no longer do so, it "gives up," dilates, weakens, and "fails." The patient is then said to have congestive heart failure. Its ability to deliver enough blood to the rest of the body decreases. Blood then backs up into the lungs and the patient becomes short of breath. The feet also swell because when the lungs are congested, blood backs up into the veins, and down the legs.

The first step in treating heart failure is to correct any ongoing condition that is causing or perpetuating it. For example, if you have high blood pressure, lower it. Try to normalize a high C-reactive protein level (see page 168). If you're diabetic, you can lower your chances of developing heart failure by using a combination of statin drugs, angiotensin-converting enzyme (ACE) inhibitors, and beta-blockers. If you've had a heart attack that has already knocked out some muscle, angioplasty or bypass surgery can open any other vessels that are ready to close up, thus preventing another heart attack. If a diseased, malformed valve is placing a burden on your heart, have it repaired or replaced.

Other specific treatments for heart failure range from drug therapy to heart transplants. Until fairly recently, the three most important and widely used medications for this purpose were digitalis, diuretics (to eliminate any retained fluid), and ACE inhibitors, whose prototype is Capoten (captopril). Although they remain effective and continue to be prescribed for most patients with heart failure, several other drugs have become available that can further prolong survival and improve the quality of life.

HERE'S WHAT'S NEW

Drugs. For many years after their discovery, beta-blockers were used mainly to lower blood pressure, slow a rapidly beating heart, correct rhythm abnormalities, and relieve angina (chest pain). Doctors were told specifically to avoid prescribing them for patients with heart failure, in the mistaken belief that they further weaken the heart muscle. But recent research has confirmed their usefulness in this condition.

There are several different beta-blockers and, for practical purposes, one is as good as another. However, several studies have shown that one in particular, Coreg (carvedilol) may be more effective than the others in treating heart failure. Equally impressive was the observation that children with severe congestive heart failure who were placed on a heart transplant waiting list sometimes could be removed from that list because they improved so much with the drug. (Coreg's greater effectiveness than other beta-blockers is limited to heart failure therapy and does not necessarily apply to other situations, such as reducing heart rate, relieving angina, and controlling rhythm disorders.)

Beta-blockers are now also routinely prescribed after a heart attack, even in the absence of congestive failure. However, they can aggravate other disorders such as chronic lung disease and arterial disease in the legs that cause pain on walking. Although beta-blockers, in conjunction with ACE inhibitors and statins, are beneficial for diabetics, they can mask the symptoms of a low blood glucose level.

Continuous positive airway pressure (CPAP). Obstructive sleep apnea—disturbed sleep patterns during which breathing stops for as long as 10 seconds—is commonly associated with coronary artery disease and high blood pressure. About 30 percent of patients with congestive heart failure also have obstructive sleep apnea.

Continuous positive airway pressure keeps airways open and prevents the breathing interruptions in people with sleep apnea. Patients are fitted with a mask attached to a machine that delivers pressurized air (not oxygen) through the nostrils.

CPAP also helps congestive heart failure that accompanies obstructive sleep apnea. Patients in whom CPAP was added to the standard heart failure treatment enjoyed better cardiac function as shown by a lower daytime systolic blood pressure (the top number), a slower heart rate, and improved pumping action of the heart.

Transplants. In addition to medication, some stunning new technological advances have emerged to help severely weakened hearts. A heart transplant is the treatment of choice, but unfortunately there are not nearly enough of them to go around. The lucky few who do receive them have a much better quality of life than those who were given them years ago, thanks to the new antirejection drugs available today. A 42-year-old woman with a human heart transplant since 1996 recently climbed the 14,000-foot Matterhorn in Switzerland. (She needed the transplant because her heart muscle was severely damaged by a virus.)

Artificial hearts. For those who need a new heart but can't wait for a transplant, new types of "artificial" hearts, or more accurately "assist devices," enable them to enjoy better quality of life. The Jarvik heart is the prototype of several others that were approved this past year. The patient's own heart is left in place, but an assist device is placed inside the left ventricle (the main chamber of the heart that does most of the pumping). It boosts the ability of the heart muscle to contract so that it can provide enough blood with each beat.

These devices were originally designed as temporary solutions for those awaiting heart transplants. However, they are functioning so well that, in many cases, heart transplants are not required. I know one such patient with an implanted Jarvik heart who says he feels better than he did before he developed heart trouble and who for the past 3 years has been hiking. (Before his surgery, he was unable to walk to the next room!)

The main problems with assist devices, besides the possibility of mechanical failure, are infection and bleeding. But these are becoming less frequent. Their track record? Some 52 percent of patients with end-stage heart failure survive for 1 year after implantation, as compared with only 25 percent treated with drug therapy. Remember, however, that these are the sickest of the sick. At 2 years, only 8 percent undergoing medical treatment alone survive, compared to nearly 25 percent of those with left ventricular assist devices. As researchers continue to solve these technical problems, the units will be more widely used.

The totally implanted heart also is being improved. Here, the patient's own heart is actually removed and replaced with an implanted device the size of a fist. Although some patients have survived a relatively short time, these hearts have not yet achieved the kind of results that should inspire you to rush to get one.

Other implant devices. Many patients with weak hearts are vulnerable to sudden death due to a rhythm disorder of the left ventricle. Most cardiologists are now convinced that these patients should receive an implantable defibrillator. This device just sits there until a life-threatening arrhythmia develops, at which point it kicks in and terminates the abnormal rhythm by shocking the heart. If everyone eligible for such a defibrillator were to receive one, there could be 200,000 fewer sudden deaths in the United States alone.

When the heart is weak, the left and right ventricles do not beat simultaneously, which reduces their efficiency. For such patients who have a specific kind of abnormality on their electrocardiogram, a "synchronizing" pacemaker can, along with the defibrillator, improve symptoms and prolong life. This pacemaker stimulates both ventricles to contract together, thus improving the cardiac output. Ask your cardiologist whether you are a candidate for such a synchronizing device.

THE BOTTOM LINE

The best way to deal with heart failure is to prevent it. However, a host of drugs is now available, the beta-blockers among them, that can greatly improve the duration and quality of life in patients with weak hearts. In addition, defibrillators, "synchronizing" pacemakers, and artificial heart assists have reduced the need for difficult-to-get heart transplants and have prolonged the lives of many people.

Surviving Cardiac Arrest

EVERY YEAR, more than 220,000 Americans suddenly collapse and die from cardiac arrest. In many cases, there's no warning. They're alive one moment and dead the next. The heart suddenly stops pumping blood; the brain (and the rest of the body) receives no nourishment and so stops functioning. Unless the arrest is treated and normal heart action restored within 4 to 6 minutes, the person dies. This lethal rhythm is not necessarily a result of weakness of the heart muscle (although arrest often occurs in people with heart failure) but instead is a disorder of the cardiac electrical system. Most patients who suffer cardiac arrest have some type of underlying heart disease, whether or not they are aware of it.

Cardiac arrest occurs in two ways. In about 25 percent of cases, the heart either slows down dramatically, beating only a few times a minute instead of the normal 60 to 80 beats per minute, or stops. In the remaining 75 percent of cases, ventricular fibrillation causes the arrest. In these cases, instead of contracting and expelling blood, the ventricles quiver ineffectively like a bag of worms and do not expel any blood.

The most effective way to deal with cardiac arrest is shock—delivered by a pacemaker to get the heart beating again if it has stopped or a defibrillator to jolt it back to normal rhythm. These machines originally were designed for use in ambulances and wherever people congregated in large numbers—airplanes, stadiums, casinos, large corporate offices, amusement parks. Personnel working in those areas were taught how to use them. It's not clear how many lives public defibrillators have actually saved. Part of the problem with the machines is that they require the immediate presence of someone who knows when and how to use them.

The next step in the defibrillator saga was the invention of a tiny unit (discussed on page 165) that is implanted in the heart of a vulnerable person to sense life-threatening rhythm and shock it back to normal.

HERE'S WHAT'S NEW

The latest advance in this area is the development and FDA approval of home defibrillators. Because 70 percent of cardiac arrests occur at home, this will have a great impact on the threat of sudden death. Although no one is immune to this catastrophe, most victims are men in their sixties with a history of heart disease. The main users of the home defibrillators are their wives.

The home defibrillator requires a doctor's prescription and costs between $2,000 and $2,500. The machine is user-friendly. It's programmed to determine whether a person actually needs the shock. So if a family member turns on the machine but the condition is, say, a stroke and not cardiac arrest, the machine will not go into the shock mode. The unit is battery-operated and beeps when the battery is low.

Although I recommend these units to selected patients who are at risk for cardiac arrest, the American Heart Association does not yet endorse their universal use. It wants more evidence that it will save lives. The National Institutes of Health has initiated a study of 7,000 people at high risk. Family members of half the subjects will be trained in CPR; families of the other half will be given defibrillators.

At the end of 4 years, the results for both groups will be tallied. In the meantime, the FDA has ordered the manufacturers to keep track of the results that are reported to them.

THE BOTTOM LINE

Home defibrillators are not for healthy people. Who wants to come home from a hard day's work and see one of these units next to the dining room table or the bed? But if you have coronary artery disease or are taking medication for an arrhythmia, ask your doctor if you are a candidate for cardiac arrest, no matter how remote the possibility. Your first choice should be an implanted defibrillator that is ready and immediately available at all times. Your next choice should be a home defibrillator.

The ABCs of C-RP

DURING THIS PAST YEAR, there has been renewed interest in the C-reactive protein (C-RP) blood test, a diagnostic tool that has been around for 65 years. Since this protein is elevated in the presence of obvious inflammation due to any cause, the C-RP test was used to diagnose and monitor the progress of infections and certain diseases that affect the immune system, such as rheumatoid arthritis. Recently, we have become aware that various parts of the body can be inflamed without causing any symptoms—no fever, no pain, no symptoms whatsoever. This silent process may indicate the presence of a life-threatening condition when it involves the lining of a blood vessel in the heart or brain. Such inflammation usually doesn't cause symptoms, but it leaves the blood vessel prone to clogging and obstruction of blood flow within it.

Inflammation, albeit silent, appears to be as important a risk factor for heart disease as are conventionally recognized ones. The clogging occurs because when any plaques already present in these inflamed vessels rupture, the resulting debris clogs the vessels and causes a heart attack or stroke. Silent inflammation explains why some people without other apparent risk factors for vascular disease and who are seemingly in good health nevertheless develop heart attacks or strokes in the prime of their lives. C-RP not only is an indicator of underlying inflammation but also is believed to stimulate the release of inflammatory substances called cytokines that further promote clotting in the arteries.

HERE'S WHAT'S NEW

C-reactive protein is now considered a better predictor of vulnerability to arteriosclerosis and its consequences than is a high LDL (bad cholesterol) level. Because someone with a high C-RP level is at twice the risk of having a heart attack or stroke, regardless of cholesterol level, knowing your C-RP level is important. It's easily determined by a blood test that costs around $15 to $20. The average reading in this country is 1.5; levels of 3 or higher are an important warning for you to take whatever steps are necessary to protect yourself.

What should you do about a high C-RP level? Will lowering it reduce your risk of vascular disease? Most doctors think so, but this has not yet been proven. A large trial of 15,000 people that began in January 2003 may provide the answer. Until then, here's what I suggest.

Rule out an infection somewhere in the body. Your doctor should make sure that you don't have an underlying infection or an autoimmune disease, such as rheumatoid arthritis or lupus, that could account for the high C-RP level.

Focus on the vascular system. You should have an electrocardiogram, a stress test, and a sonogram of the carotid arteries in the neck to look for evidence of arteriosclerosis. I also sometimes order an ultrafast CT scan of the chest or an equivalent test to identify calcium deposits in and around the coronary arteries.

Control your risk factors. If your C-RP level is high, identify and correct any other risk factors you may have. However, even if you have none, check your blood pressure; follow a diet low in saturated fat and rich in oily fish; eat lots of fruit, vegetables, and whole grains; exercise regularly; try to achieve ideal weight; and if you smoke, quit.

Consider taking a statin drug. The following is a key recommendation, regardless of your cholesterol level. Besides normalizing blood fats, statin drugs such as Lipitor (atorvastatin) and Pravachol (pravastatin) also reduce inflammation, thus stabilizing any plaques in your coronary arteries and reducing the likelihood of their clotting. They have been shown to lower C-RP by 15 to 25 percent. A recent study shows that high doses of statin drugs (80 milligrams of Lipitor) decreased C-RP levels by almost 30 percent in patients with type 2 diabetes (who are especially vulnerable to vascular disease).

Have a drink. Adults who drank three to four glasses of beer with dinner lowered their C-RP levels by about 35 percent after 3 weeks, presumably because of the anti-inflammatory properties of alcohol. As far as I'm concerned, that's a lot of beer, with or without dinner! My advice is to have a cocktail or a glass or two of wine with your evening meal—but no more than that. More is not better, especially if you'll be driving later on.

Get help from a pill. In another study, people who took a multivitamin also dropped their C-RP levels (and lowered their homocysteine levels as well—see page 171). The researchers in this particular study believe that this beneficial effect was a result of vitamins B and C. (However, several other studies have found no benefit from multivitamins overall.) The antibiotic Vibramycin (doxycycline), widely used to treat gum disease, was recently found to lower C-RP levels by nearly 50 percent in patients with acute heart attacks. A daily aspirin or other nonsteroidal anti-inflammatory drug (taken after meals) also should be standard therapy for a high C-RP level.

THE BOTTOM LINE

Make sure the C-RP test is part of your routine physical. If your level is elevated, start immediately to control your risk factors and ask your doctor about taking a statin drug, regardless of your cholesterol level, especially if you're diabetic.

If your cholesterol level is normal or low, should you have a C-RP test anyway? You bet! Although the American Heart Association and the Centers for Disease Control and Prevention recommend routine C-RP testing only for people at risk of heart disease, in my own practice I do it for virtually every adult patient. Many people have heart attacks and strokes even with no risk factors other than high C-RP levels.

What if your cholesterol level is high and you know you're already at increased risk for vascular disease? Should you have the C-RP test anyway? I believe it's a good idea because if both cholesterol and C-RP levels are high, you are at substantially greater risk and should be more aggressive about preventive measures.

How (And Why) to Lower Your Homocysteine

HOMOCYSTEINE is a protein by-product of normal metabolism. Its levels can be measured in the blood. When they're elevated, you're at increased risk for a heart attack, high blood pressure, stroke, and blood clots in the deep veins of the legs. The upper limit of normal depends on the laboratory performing the test but should be less than 15 micromol per liter.

HERE'S WHAT'S NEW

Besides the risks noted above, new evidence suggests that a high homocysteine blood level is also associated with sudden death, especially in diabetics, and twice the risk of Alzheimer's disease, regardless of age or sex.

In people who lack vitamin B, usually because they don't get enough in their diets, homocysteine levels rise. They can be reduced by 25 to 35 percent with a combination of B vitamins—specifically folic acid and vitamins B_6 and B_{12}. These vitamins break down homocysteine, and prevent its accumulation. (Folic acid alone will lower homocysteine levels but not as much as when combined with the other two B vitamins.)

One study found that patients who took these supplements for 6 months after undergoing angioplasty were 32 percent less likely to suffer another blockage, have a heart attack, or die during the following year. However, another more recent study revealed no benefit from lowering it. In other words, homocysteine may simply be a marker for heart disease and stroke. Its elevation should prompt you to aggressively control all other risk factors.

As with many health breakthroughs, these findings are not without debate. New research suggests that high doses of folic acid may trigger cell overgrowth in the coronary arteries and actually predispose the arteries to early closure after angioplasty. Because this has been observed only with high doses of folic acid, you should limit your intake of folic acid to 1 milligram a day.

THE BOTTOM LINE

If your homocysteine level is high, you should take 1 milligram of folic acid a day (current U.S. dietary recommendations call for only 0.4 milligram) as well as 10 milligrams of vitamin B_6 and 400 micrograms (0.4 milligram) of vitamin B_{12} even though the benefit of

doing so has been questioned. You should also have your homocysteine levels checked two or three times a year.

Eating foods rich in the B vitamins (leafy green vegetables, low-
fat dairy products, citrus fruits and juices, whole wheat bread, cereals,
and dry beans) is also useful, but getting the right amount in the diet
is more difficult than taking a fixed, adequate dose in a pill every
morning. So even if you decide to go the diet route, take a multivitamin containing folic acid every morning just to be sure. I do not believe the last word on homocysteine has been spoken.

Even Newer Tests

IT'S INTERESTING to look back at how our understanding of the risk
factors of cardiovascular disease has evolved over the years. When I
graduated from medical school, the only definite one was a family
history of the disease. If either of your parents, one or more siblings,
or any other immediate blood relatives had cardiovascular problems
at an early age, you were considered vulnerable.

As we continue to learn more about how and why arteries become
diseased and interfere with blood flow to various organs, we realize
that there are several other indicators of vulnerability to premature
heart disease and stroke. These include cigarette smoking, lack of regular physical exercise, overweight, diabetes, high blood pressure, and
abnormal blood fat levels, including cholesterol levels. A person's risk
profile is now largely based on an assessment of all these risk factors.

Every now and then, however, men and women who do not fit
into any of these categories are affected by vascular disease at an early
age. For example, between one-third and one-half of heart attacks
occur in people with normal cholesterol levels. Doctors have been
searching for ways to identify these patients so as to forestall their
disease. Recently, we have begun to recognize the importance of

silent inflammation of the blood vessels (when the blood vessel lining is inflamed and prone to clogging but causes no acute symptoms) as yet another marker and contributing factor to premature vascular disease. As mentioned earlier, C-reactive protein and homocysteine levels, a reflection of such inflammation, have now been shown to predict vulnerability to heart attack and stroke more accurately than even the much vaunted "bad" cholesterol (LDL). Doctors are now evaluating ways of reducing high C-RP readings in an attempt to reduce the risk of heart disease.

HERE'S WHAT'S NEW

Several large clinical trials have indicated that the level of apolipoprotein (Apo for short) in the blood is a predictor of heart disease.

Apolipoproteins are tiny fat particles—of which there are several varieties (the best known are ApoA1 and ApoB)—that circulate in the blood. According to studies published in the medical journal *The Lancet*, a high ApoB level or a high ApoB:ApoA1 ratio is a very sensitive indicator of vulnerability to vascular disease. Researchers believe that doctors should now routinely measure these apolipoproteins in patients at risk. The term *apolipoprotein* sounds complicated, but this test is actually easier to perform than a cholesterol screen and doesn't require the patient to fast beforehand.

Finally, the FDA has approved yet another test, this one specifically recommended for those with low or normal cholesterol levels who are considered at risk for vascular disease because of other risk factors. Called the PLAC test, it measures an enzyme known as PLA2 that is active in the inflammatory process of the lining of the small arteries. Patients with high concentrations of this enzyme have twice the risk of heart attacks, despite low levels of LDL cholesterol. The cost of this latest test is about $16, which is about the same as the C-RP analysis.

THE BOTTOM LINE

New evidence suggests that every routine checkup of adult males and females should include tests for vulnerability to premature heart disease. This evaluation should consist of a careful family history, complete physical examination, electrocardiogram at rest and/or after exercise, and blood analyses for levels of total cholesterol, LDL, HDL, homocysteine, blood glucose, and C-RP. It now appears that looking at ApoB (ideally, the ApoB:ApoA1 ratio) as well as the PLAC test can provide even greater predictability of premature heart disease.

WHAT THE DOCTOR ORDERED?

THE FISH OIL DEBATE ● Several studies over the years have suggested that eating fish, especially oily ones, reduces the risk of heart attack. The omega-3 fatty acids that fish contain lower blood pressure a little, reduce levels of other harmful fats, inhibit the growth of artery-blocking plaques, prevent the formation of arterial blood clots, and decrease the incidence of heart disease in diabetics. In addition to protecting the heart, omega-3s are also good for the eyes and reduce airway constriction spasm in asthmatics as well.

During the past year several conflicting reports have emerged about how much fish one should eat. Some also emphasize the potential danger of the mercury content in certain fish; others are less concerned. Unless you read *all* these studies, you may not get a balanced view of what is good for you—and what may be bad.

HERE'S WHAT'S NEW ● Originally, the American Heart Association (AHA) recommended two servings a week of oily fish, both for healthy individuals and for people with heart disease. They then revised this advice because several large clinical trials found that individuals with heart disease need more than two servings. The AHA now recommends eating fish such as mackerel, lake trout, herring, sardines, tuna, and salmon *every day* to get the required 1 gram of the necessary omega-3 fatty acids. You may need even more if your blood triglyceride levels are elevated. (But then tell your doctor how much you're eating, because eating too much fish may interfere with the clotting mechanism of the blood and cause excessive bleeding.)

The AHA recommends that healthy people continue to eat two servings of oily fish a week. Pregnant women, nursing mothers, and children should avoid mackerel, tilefish, swordfish, tuna, and shark. These fish contain high levels of mercury, dioxins, and PCBs, chemicals that are potentially hazardous to children's nervous systems. However, cooked shellfish, canned light tuna, and smaller ocean fish are safe. The latest blockbuster news about eating most types of fish during pregnancy is that the mercury levels in most fish may not affect the fetus least of all neurologically. However, researchers still caution that the above-mentioned varieties containing the highest amounts of mercury should probably be avoided.

So far, so good. But hot on the heels of the AHA advice there appeared two conflicting reports in the *New England Journal of Medicine*. One stated that mercury levels in men who'd had heart attacks were 15 percent higher than those in healthy men. Researchers believe that the toxic effects of mercury in fish not only cancel out the cardiovascular benefits of the omega-3 fatty acids but actually make matters worse. However, not everyone agrees. A second study in the same journal found that there was no correlation between eating fish, mercury levels, and heart attacks. What's a consumer to think?

Meanwhile, studies continue to find even more benefits from fish. One report in the *Journal of the American Medical Association* concluded that men who consumed 3 to 5 ounces of fish only one to three times a month were 43 percent less likely to have a stroke during the next 12 years!

There appears to be yet another important reason to eat lots of oily fish like salmon, tuna, and bluefish—at least twice a week. The fatty acids they contain prevent life-threatening cardiac arrhythmias. These fatty acids, which are stored in the cell membranes of the heart, control the entry and exit of chemicals such as calcium that can predispose the heart to dangerous rhythm disturbances. The researchers are so impressed with the protective action of the fatty acids against sudden death that they are recommending that people take omega-3 supplements, because the necessary 1 gram a day may not be available through diet alone.

Another study, reported in the *British Medical Journal*, looked at the effects of regular intake of fish in more than 1,600 people older than age 68 living in southwest France. Researchers found that those who ate fish regularly for at least 7 years had a substantially lower incidence of Alzheimer's disease. Anyone who had eaten fish at least once a week derived some benefit, but the more fish they consumed, the better off they were.

But wait! It isn't as simple as that. Just eating fish is not enough. How you prepare it is also important, according to a study reported in the journal *Circulation*. Baking or broiling is the way to go. In a large, population-based study of adults older than 65, fried fish and fish sandwiches offered no beneficial cardiac effects.

THE BOTTOM LINE • Eating fish is clearly good for you. Despite all the warnings about mercury, I still believe that if you have heart disease, the more fish you eat—especially oily ones such as salmon and tuna—the better. And if you don't like fish or can't afford it, buy omega-3 supplements to make sure you consume at least 1 gram a day. OmegaBrite, Solgar, and Twinlab are reliable brands. Unless properly made, the oil can become rancid.

Pregnant women should limit consumption of ocean-going fish that contain the highest concentrations of mercury, including mackerel, tilefish, swordfish, tuna, and shark, although canned light tuna is safe.

Finally, whatever fish you end up eating, make sure you don't fry it! ●

Mammograms to Detect Heart Disease

THIS YEAR one of the most hallowed medical theories refuted by new research findings was that menopausal women should take hormone replacement therapy (HRT). It not only fails to protect against vascular diseases but also may increase its risk (see page 243).

The value and cost-effectiveness of another time-honored practice, the regular mammogram, was also for a time questioned (see page 46). After much debate, the consensus appears to be that, properly interpreted (something you shouldn't take for granted, because diagnostic skills vary greatly among radiologists), mammograms are useful and every woman should have one regularly starting just before menopause or soon after (that is, between ages 40 and 50).

HERE'S WHAT'S NEW

Besides finding cancer in the breast before a woman or her doctor can feel it, mammograms can also indicate vulnerability to heart disease early in the game. That's because the x-rays beamed at the breasts also can identify calcifications in the coronary arteries. Women with these calcifications are 20 percent more likely to develop heart disease.

THE BOTTOM LINE

Do not have a mammogram just to look for evidence of heart disease. However, when the radiologist reports the findings to you, ask whether he or she happened to see any calcifications in your coronary arteries. If they were present (and that's more likely in women older than age 60), let your doctor know. You may then be advised to undergo other tests to clarify their significance because, according to researchers at the Mayo Clinic, there's a one in five chance that coronary calcifications detected this way reflect underlying heart disease.

When to Say No to Antioxidants

THERE IS WIDESPREAD BELIEF that antioxidants prevent heart disease, reduce its severity, or both. The most popular antioxidants in the United States are vitamins C and E and beta-carotene.

HERE'S WHAT'S NEW

Recent research indicates that most adult diabetics should take a cholesterol-lowering drug, such as a statin, even if their cholesterol levels are normal and they don't have heart disease. These medications were originally recommended only for people with high cholesterol levels. However, in a new study of 20,000 diabetics, those taking a 40-milligram tablet of Zocor (simvastatin)—one of several available statins—had a 25 percent lower risk of subsequent cardiovascular events such as a heart attack.

New findings by researchers at the University of Washington may surprise you. The scientists evaluated 160 people with heart disease who were taking cholesterol-lowering drugs (Zocor and niacin). Half of them were also on one or more antioxidants. After 3 years, the incidence of new vascular disease—including death, stroke, another heart attack, or the need for angioplasty or bypass surgery—

was much lower (3 percent) among those who took the anticholesterol medication *without* the antioxidants. The subjects receiving both antioxidants *and* cholesterol-lowering drugs experienced a 14 percent incidence of these events—almost four times as many as the others.

In a British study of 20,000 patients taking antioxidants alone (that is, without cholesterol-lowering drugs), the antioxidants had no effect whatsoever on the incidence of vascular disease.

Now here's the clincher. In the most recent evaluation of the effectiveness of antioxidants on the cardiovascular system, researchers at the Cleveland Clinic Foundation analyzed the results from 15 studies involving 220,000 people, most of whom were either very vulnerable to heart and vascular disease or already had it. All of them had been followed for as long as 12 years, enough time to tell whether something works or doesn't. The study found that vitamin E and beta-carotene, alone or together, did not improve a vascular status. In fact, beta-carotene alone actually *increased* the risk of cardiovascular disease as well as death from any cause.

Staunch believers in these vitamins are now suggesting that they help prevent vascular disease in *healthy* people, but not in those already affected. That's an interesting possibility, and only time and further studies will yield the answer. As for me personally, I have stopped taking antioxidant supplements but I continue to eat foods that contain them. That means at least five servings of fresh fruits and vegetables every day.

THE BOTTOM LINE

Most people with heart disease who take a cholesterol-lowering drug should avoid antioxidant supplements. Though antioxidants reduce the incidence of upper-respiratory tract infections in diabetics, those on a cholesterol-lowering drug should not take these supplements, especially if they already have some evidence of vascular disease. It's better to have a cold than a heart attack!

However, if you are at risk for colon cancer because of a strong family history, and you are also a nonsmoker and nondrinker, the antioxidant beta-carotene may decrease your chances of developing this malignancy (see page 84).

Drink Wisely—Or Not at All

WE'VE KNOWN FOR SEVERAL YEARS that alcohol in moderation protects men and post-menopausal women against heart disease. It probably does so by raising blood levels of HDL (the "good" cholesterol) and certain cardioprotective enzymes and proteins. Every now and then you'll read that a particular form of alcohol is more effective than others—be it beer, white wine, or red wine—the latter presumably because of the resveratrol content in the skin of grapes. (Resveratrol is a chemical with many different properties, but it's best known as an antioxidant.)

HERE'S WHAT'S NEW

The latest studies relating to alcohol's effect on the heart emphasize that it isn't the kind of alcohol you drink or whether you take it with a meal that's important. The key appears to be *how much* and *how often* you imbibe.

In a 12-year study of 38,000 male health professionals ages 40 to 75, none of whom had heart disease, researchers found that those who consumed any type of alcoholic beverage 3 or more days a week reduced their risk of a subsequent heart attack by about one-third, as compared with those who drank less alcohol. Two drinks a day appeared to be the optimal amount; more was not better.

THE BOTTOM LINE

If you enjoy moderate social drinking, continue to do so. But don't ignore other risk factors, including weight, smoking, cholesterol levels, and exercise. Most important, don't interpret this new information as a prescription to start drinking if you've never done so before, because despite these findings, alcohol hurts more than it helps. As one editorial in the *New England Journal of Medicine* put it, if alcohol were a new drug, the FDA would probably not approve it. Its many toxic effects and complications—the risk of addiction; the violence and accidents that occur with its use; the damage to the liver, gastrointestinal tract, brain, kidneys, and even the heart in some cases—far outweigh its benefits. There are other, more effective and less risky ways to reduce your risk of heart disease.

Angioplasty and the New Stents

IT WASN'T LONG AGO that the only way for doctors to get blood flowing through a clogged coronary artery was to perform a bypass operation. Many thousands of these surgeries were done throughout the country, with excellent results. They are still being performed, but much less frequently. That's because angioplasty, the art of ballooning open these blood vessels, has been so successfully refined. In my own practice, for every patient I refer for a bypass operation, I send 10 for angioplasty.

Angioplasty has become even more successful since the development of stents, little mesh "sleeves" that are placed inside the artery to keep them open after blood flow has been restored. These stents have further reduced the chances of clots reforming after the angioplasty balloon compresses the obstructing plaques against the artery wall.

HERE'S WHAT'S NEW

Although stenting has reduced the incidence of reclosure after ballooning, it has nevertheless remained at about 30 percent, especially in smaller coronary arteries in which blood flow is not as brisk.

In April 2003, a new stent was released that has lowered the incidence of closure to less than 10 percent. It is coated with the drug rapamycin. When applied to the stents, rapamycin prevents those changes in the wall of the artery that ultimately lead to clot formation. This new technology will further reduce the need for coronary bypass surgery.

THE BOTTOM LINE

If you have angina or other symptoms of coronary artery narrowing, an angiogram will determine the extent and location of the blockage. In many cases, these arteries can be ballooned open with angioplasty and then stented. Ideally, you should have a rapamycin-coated stent. Unfortunately, because of its higher cost, this stent is not always made available. I am told that some insurance carriers will pay for it only after the older devices have failed. If you have any say in the matter, insist on a rapamycin-coated stent the first time around to keep your ballooned artery open.

The Latest Aspirin News

IT'S A RARE MEDICAL MEETING where some researcher fails to come up with yet another benefit of aspirin for a malady (heart disease, cancer, pain—you name it). What started as a simple over-the-counter pill to reduce fever and control mild pain has evolved into what is arguably the most versatile drug available to mankind. It not only reduces elevated temperature and eases soreness but also helps prevent strokes, heart attacks, and various cancers. And that's probably only the beginning of the aspirin saga.

With regard to aspirin's role in vascular disease, we have known for years that it protects men who are at high risk for developing vascular problems (this is called primary prevention). An aspirin a day also reduces the risk of a second heart attack or stroke in men who've already had one (secondary prevention). Aspirin interferes with blood clotting by acting on blood platelets so they don't clump together and form clots in the arteries. This is why someone taking aspirin for any reason bleeds more easily and why it is usually discontinued before an operation.

HERE'S WHAT'S NEW

Aspirin is not just for men. Researchers always assumed, but never proved, that women also benefit from aspirin. Now, scientists at Miami's Mount Sinai Medical Center and Heart Institute have found that aspirin does reduce the risk of a first heart attack in high-risk individuals of *both* sexes. This conclusion is based on an analysis of results from five different studies. Some 55,000 subjects, 11,000 of them women, were divided into two groups—those who took daily aspirin (anywhere from 81 to 325 milligrams) and those who didn't. The aspirin protected both women and men, providing an overall reduction of 32 percent in the rate of heart attacks, strokes, and other vascular events.

High cholesterol level reduces aspirin's benefit. Here's a new twist. Recent research from the University of Maryland suggests that in order for aspirin to exert its protective effect on the cardiovascular system, the cholesterol level must be normal. When it's elevated, aspirin does not as efficiently prevent blood platelets from clumping and forming clots.

Low-dose and coated tablets aren't as effective. Two new studies have appeared, one of which, if true, will disappoint many users of aspirin, including me. Doctors running the stroke program at Northwestern Memorial Hospital in Chicago are suggesting that low-dose aspirin (81 milligrams), the so-called children's aspirin, is not nearly as effective in preventing the abnormal blood clotting that leads to heart attack and stroke as are higher strengths. Neither are the coated tablets.

The researchers observed that more than half of the 250 subjects who were taking aspirin (either low-dose aspirin or coated tablets) experienced no anticlotting benefits and developed heart attacks and strokes. Platelets were affected in only 44 percent of those taking the 81-milligram dose of aspirin, as compared with 72 percent of those on the 325-milligram dose. That's a big difference. As far as coating was concerned, it had no impact on platelets in 65 percent of cases, whereas the uncoated pills reduced clotting in 75 percent.

Aspirin shouldn't be combined with ibuprofen. Researchers in the United Kingdom found that combining aspirin with ibuprofen (such as Motrin) on a regular basis also interferes with its anticlotting properties. Many people, especially the elderly, use these two drugs together. They take aspirin for protection against vascular disease and ibuprofen or a similar drug to ease their aches and pains. In a well-conducted study, researchers found that those who took aspirin with ibuprofen on a regular basis were twice as likely to die of cardiovascular disease as people on aspirin alone.

THE BOTTOM LINE

Whether you're male or female, if you're at high risk for having a heart attack or stroke, take an aspirin every day and make sure your cholesterol level is within normal limits. If this advice were heeded, it's estimated that there would be 350,000 fewer heart attacks and other vascular events every year.

For the time being, until another study comes out refuting the above findings, you're better off taking the full-strength tablet (325 milligrams) of uncoated aspirin. However, if you are prone to stomach irritation or are a senior citizen, the larger dose may present a problem, so check with your doctor.

What the Doctor Ordered?

TAKE ASPIRIN, SPARE YOUR GUT ● Even the 81-milligram low-dose aspirin, including the enteric-coated form, can irritate your stomach and be more likely to cause gastrointestinal bleeding if you have a stomach ulcer.

HERE'S WHAT'S NEW ● The latest research indicates that stomachache from aspirin may be due to something other than the drug—namely a bacterium called *Helicobacter pylori*. Researchers in Japan found that animals experimentally infected with *H. pylori* and given aspirin were much more likely to develop irritation of the stomach lining than those taking aspirin but free of *H. pylori*.

In humans, this bug may cause stomach ulcers (with and without aspirin on board) and has also been linked to gastric cancer.

Doctors at the Chinese University of Hong Kong who studied several hundred patients found that eliminating *H. pylori* with the appropriate antibiotics allowed them to take aspirin with few, if any, of the side effects they'd previously had (abdominal pain, gas, and indigestion).

THE BOTTOM LINE ● If you must take aspirin regularly and find it irritates your stomach, or if you have a peptic ulcer, ask your doctor to check you for *H. pylori*. It's easy to do with either a breath test or a blood analysis. If you test positive, you can eradicate the organism by taking an antibiotic for 10 to 14 days. It's well worth it. Not only is there a good chance that you'll be able to take the aspirin you need but you may also reduce your risk of developing stomach cancer sometime in the future. And here's an extra bonus: If you have bad breath for which your dentist can find no cause, it just may come from your stomach—if any *H. pylori* is present. Getting rid of this bacterium may have you smelling very sweet, even when you exhale (see page 35).

It's also a good idea to be tested for *H. pylori* if you are taking a nonsteroidal anti-inflammatory drug such as ibuprofen to relieve chronic pain. If you are infected, eradicating the organism will minimize stomach irritation caused by these medications. However, you still may need to take an acid-reducing drug such as Prilosec (omeprazole) to further reduce your risk of bleeding.

HEMORRHOIDS

· · · · · · · · · ·

A Pain in the Butt

IF YOU NEED PROOF about the prevalence and importance of hemorrhoids in our country, ponder on this statistic: The second most commonly shoplifted item from our nation's pharmacies is Preparation H, arguably the best-known and most widely used hemorrhoidal cream in the United States!

The rectum has a network of veins which, when engorged, enlarged, and often inflamed, are called hemorrhoids (affectionately known as "piles"). They can be external (at the anal opening), visible to anyone who's looking, or internal (at the origin of the anal canal inside the rectum) where they can be felt but not seen. Hemorrhoids are not contagious, they never become cancerous, and *everyone* has them at some time or other.

What is it that turns these harmless little rectal veins into nasty, big, painful, bleeding piles? The major causes are constipation and diarrhea, repeated heavy lifting, coughing, standing or sitting for long periods of time, overweight, and pregnancy. And then there's anal intercourse.

Thankfully, hemorrhoids don't always cause symptoms, but they do act up from time to time in one of every two Americans of both genders, usually between the ages of 20 and 50. When they do, they cause pain, itching, and bleeding.

HERE'S WHAT'S NEW

Unfortunately, there's little that's groundbreaking in the prevention or treatment of hemorrhoids. But as this is a problem some patients *still* find too embarrassing to speak to their doctors about, the tried-and-true strategies bear repeating here.

For prevention:

Keep "moving." Since constipation is the handmaiden of hemorrhoids, it's very important to respond as soon as possible to nature's signal.

Don't strain. Do your reading somewhere other than on the toilet.

Follow the right diet. Eat lots of fiber (whole-grain breads, 3 to 4 tablespoons of bran per day), cereals, bran muffins, beans, fresh fruit (especially plums, apricots, and apples), stewed or canned fruit (prunes, figs), fruit juices (orange, prune, fig), vegetables (celery, lettuce, spinach, turnips, carrots, cabbage), brown rice, nuts, and lots and lots of water (2 quarts or more per day).

Cut down on caffeine and alcohol. Both of these tend to make the stool dry and hard.

Avoid laxatives. They can be irritating.

Get enough exercise. It helps prevent constipation and also improves the tone of the muscles supporting the rectal area.

Lose weight. The extra pounds place more pressure on the rectal area.

When hemorrhoids become troublesome, resting your feet on a low stool while you're sitting on the toilet makes it less painful to move your bowels. Afterwards, use moistened toilet paper, and pat, don't wipe vigorously. For relief, apply ice to the anal area. Some patients prefer a wet, warm tea bag or a witch hazel compress. Apply any of these for about 10 minutes three or four times a day. Unfortunately, that's not easy to do on the job. When you get home, sit in 8 to 10 inches of water for 15 to 20 minutes at least a couple of times before you go to bed.

It's easier said than done, but try not to scratch. Avoid narcotics such as codeine, which, though they relieve pain, can cause constipation. Stay with a nonprescription medication such as a nonsteroidal anti-inflammatory drug (Advil, Aleve) two or three times a day. Several over-the-counter topical agents—ointments, creams, and suppositories—can provide relief from the pain and itching of hemorrhoids. The best known are zinc oxide ointments such as Preparation H, and Anusol-HC cream with 1 percent hydrocortisone to reduce the swelling, burning, and itching of external hemorrhoids. The same formulation comes in suppository form for internal swelling and discomfort.

Straining increases pressure on the rectal veins. A stool softener such as docusate, a stimulant to bowel contraction such as Senokot, or a bulking agent containing psyllium seed, such as Metamucil, Konsyl, and Citrucel (all of which you can buy without a prescription) will keep the movements soft and easily passed. Buy a doughnut-shaped cushion on which to sit for long hours at your desk or in your car.

If hemorrhoid symptoms become more severe despite all the measures described above; here are some other treatment options:

- Internal hemorrhoids that bleed or protrude after bowel movement can be tied off at their base by your doctor using a small rubber band that cuts off their blood supply. The rubber band and the hemorrhoids both fall off in about 7 days.

- Bleeding hemorrhoids that do not protrude can be injected with a chemical that scars them (sclerotherapy).

- Hemorrhoids can be coagulated (clotted) by infrared photocoagulation. (Unlike the other techniques, this one may require more than one treatment, but it is relatively painless.)

- Lasers direct a high-intensity light beam at the hemorrhoid, cauterizing or coagulating it. Laser therapy is expensive, and it can hurt just as much as surgery to remove the hemorrhoids.

- You may have no choice but an operation if clots keep forming in your external hemorrhoids, or if the rubber band ligation and other methods fail to prevent the internal ones from slipping out of the rectum (prolapsing).

THE BOTTOM LINE

Several topical medications and suppositories can alleviate pain, itching, and bleeding. Make sure that the bleeding is not masking a tumor in the bowel. Blood in the stool, regardless of whether or not you have hemorrhoids, should always be investigated further.

If home remedies fail to control the pain or stop the bleeding, several measures are available. My first choice among all of these is the rubber-band ligation, which is easy, quick, and painless. However, surgical removal is the most predictable way to solve a recurring hemorrhoid problem. A colorectal specialist, not a primary doctor, should perform these procedures.

HEPATITIS

* * * * * * * * *

Live Better with a Healthy Liver

THE LIVER IS A CRITICAL ORGAN that performs a host of functions that keep us alive. Too bad it doesn't beat, breathe, or pee like other organs; we all might take better care of it. The liver is our refinery. It converts the chicken, potatoes, cheese, and carrots we eat into protein, calcium, iron, fat, and vitamins—storing those you don't need right away for a "rainy day." You also can thank your liver for mopping up toxic waste such as naturally occurring bacteria, harmful by-products of everyday bodily functions, and the alcohol from too many martinis. That just scratches the surface of what this amazing organ does each day.

Although any bug or parasite can infect the liver, right now, viral hepatitis is the big one in our part of the world. The three most common hepatitis viruses are A, B, and C. They can make you very sick with jaundice, nausea, vomiting, loss of appetite, insomnia, and abdominal swelling and pain. In the cases of hepatitis B and especially C, they can also kill you.

There are as many ways to contract hepatitis as there are to interact with other human beings or the environment. Hepatitis A virus (HAV) can infect you when you eat either cooked or uncooked food, as well as when you drink water contaminated with the feces of an infected person. You can also "catch" it from close contact with someone who's infected. Hepatitis B (HBV) is transmitted not only from blood but also a variety of other body fluids—semen, vaginal discharge, tears, saliva, and breast milk. Hepatitis C (HCV), one of the most serious and common blood-borne infections in the United States, can be spread through sharing contaminated needles, razors, toothbrushes, and other personal items, as well as from sexual partners. It can also be passed from pregnant women to their babies.

HERE'S WHAT'S NEW

There is a vaccine that prevents HAV. If you're a health care worker and vulnerable, a man who has sex with other men, a substance abuser in the habit of sharing needles, or a traveler visiting some place where the hygiene leaves much to be desired, you should have the shot. I also recommend HAV vaccination to all my patients with other forms of liver disease that would be aggravated if they were to become infected with HAV. It's also a good idea for Alaskans and other Native Americans, whose incidence of HAV infection is high, to have their children vaccinated at 2 years of age.

The HAV vaccine is not a live virus and so can't cause the disease. Adults over the age of 18 need two shots, 6 to 12 months apart. Children and adolescents should receive the vaccine in three doses; the second about 1 month after the first and the third 6 to 12 months later. If you've been exposed to the virus in the past 14 days and have not been previously vaccinated, you should receive a shot of gamma globulin, a preparation of antibodies that provides short-term protection. Doing so may prevent the disease or reduce its severity. Hepatitis A rarely kills or makes you sick over the long term.

Hepatitis B is a different story. Although 90 percent of those infected recover completely, the 10 percent who do develop chronic HBV can become seriously ill or die. Should you contract HBV, ask your doctor about Epivir-HBV (lamivudine) and interferon alfa-2b, the two drugs that have been approved for the treatment of this disease. They can protect the liver in about one-fourth of the cases. (I'm hedging on using the word "cure," because some patients respond for a while, then relapse.) Several other medications are currently being evaluated as well.

There's also a safe and effective vaccine available for HBV that everyone, including newborns, should get since we're all vulnerable to the disease. You need three shots over a 6-month period. Don't bother asking for the vaccine if you were previously infected. You're already protected against re-infection.

If you have recently been exposed to hepatitis B or have been accidentally stuck with an infected or questionable needle, you should receive hepatitis B immune globulin within 24 hours and no later than 7 days after exposure. Then get a repeat dose 30 days later. You should also have the vaccine, because it adds long-term protection to the short-term benefit of the immune globulin.

Although we can treat the symptoms of hepatitis C once they appear, there is no predictable way to prevent the disease from becoming chronic. However, even if you have no symptoms, you should consider the antiviral therapy that's currently available. You may be one of the lucky ones who respond. Treatment regimens vary somewhat. Most specialists advise PEGASYS (pegylated interferon) once a week, as well as two capsules a day of the antiviral drug Rebetol (ribavirin), continued for 6 to 12 months. This program has resulted in a sustained response in more than half the patients treated. There is no vaccine for HCV, but you should be immunized against A and B.

THE BOTTOM LINE

HAV is almost always a benign disease that does not hurt the liver over the long term. However, you may feel lousy for weeks. Unlike hepatitis A, hepatitis B is potentially serious. Although the great majority of those who develop it do recover, some do not. HCV is a silent killer. Unlike A and B, it quietly destroys your liver over the years. You should seek appropriate medical treatment for each of these viral infections.

HIGH BLOOD
PRESSURE

· · · · · · · · ·

What Your Reading Really Means

CONSIDER THIS: Hypertension (high blood pressure) is a major killer and crippler in this country. More than 50 million Americans older than age 6 (this is not a typo—kids get it too) have high blood pressure. That's about one in every four of us. The incidence increases with age, so by age 75, two out of every three people are afflicted with it. Unfortunately, about one-third of those who have it don't know it. Among those who do, half are treated inadequately and continue to live with dangerously high blood pressure that ultimately weakens their hearts, clogs arteries throughout their bodies, and predisposes them to heart attacks, strokes, blindness, and kidney failure.

Despite this danger, there is little agreement among laypeople (and even doctors) about what constitutes high blood pressure. Ask around. You'll find some people who believe that a normal systolic pressure (the top number) is 100 plus your age. Others say the reading should be below 140/90. Many opine that the diastolic pressure (the lower figure) should not exceed 80. To further complicate matters, some "experts" insist that the top number doesn't matter and only the bottom one is important.

When I was a medical student, we were taught that numbers were not important and that we were not to treat anyone as long as they had no complaints such as headache or nosebleed!

Well, we've come a long way since then, but a great deal of controversy still exists. For example, some doctors insist that even when the pressure is "high" by any definition, the significance of the elevation depends on where the reading was obtained—at home on your own cuff, on a machine in a supermarket, or by the doctor. Patients will tell me, "You make me nervous, doctor. My pressure is always normal when I take it in the drugstore or the supermarket. Haven't you heard of white coat hypertension?" So I put on a blue coat and record their pressure. The reading is usually unchanged. It's even high when my nurse, in her *blue* uniform, records it. So they conclude that it must be the surroundings, not me. And so on.

Once everyone (patient, doctor, and supermarket blood pressure machine) has agreed that a reading is high, the next question is how best to treat it. Some specialists advocate exercise, weight loss, and reducing salt intake for as long as it takes to get results. Others say that time is of the essence and that medication should be started as soon as the diagnosis is made. When everyone concerned has decided that it's time to take medication, a whole new debate begins as to what drugs to use. It's like a medical tower of Babel.

HERE'S WHAT'S NEW

Someone finally decided to clear up the confusion. In 2003, the Joint National Committee on Prevention, Detection, Evaluation, and Treatment of High Blood Pressure met in Washington and released its seventh report to the nation. Let's hope that its conclusions and recommendations will clarify the ambiguity about this major affliction of mankind.

Here are the new criteria, in a nutshell.

Normal: Any reading *less than* 120/80.

Prehypertension: Blood pressure readings between 120–139/80–89, though strictly speaking "normal," are considered to be *prehypertensive*. These levels do not require medication, but you should start making certain lifestyle changes such as eliminating risk factors that contribute to future cardiovascular disease—smoking, excess weight, poor diet (you should be eating less saturated fat and more fruits and vegetables), lack of regular exercise, and too much dietary salt.

Stage 1 hypertension: Blood pressure readings of 140–159/90–99 call for treatment usually with only one drug, preferably a diuretic ("water pill"). However, if along with stage 1 hypertension you also have a weak heart, abnormal cardiac rhythm, a valve problem, or some kidney disorder in which a diuretic might be harmful, it may be better to start with a medication from another antihypertensive drug class, such as an angiotensin-converting enzyme (ACE) inhibitor, angiotensin-receptor blocker (ARB), beta-blocker, or calcium channel blocker.

Stage 2 hypertension (there is no longer a stage 3): Readings of 160/100 or higher almost always require two or more antihypertensives, but start with one. You never know; it may be enough. Preferably, it should be a "water pill," which is not only the safest but the cheapest, too.

THE BOTTOM LINE

I believe these recommendations are sound, and I expect that most doctors will follow them. Basically, 140/90 remains the goal for most people being treated for hypertension. However, if you're diabetic or have chronic kidney disease, your pressure should be kept below 130/80.

After age 50, the systolic pressure is a much more important risk factor than the diastolic pressure. Keep it below 140. This is a major shift from opinions of yesteryear, when systolic pressure was ignored and the importance of diastolic pressure was emphasized.

Monitor your pressure regularly. There is no guarantee that even an ideal reading such as 115/75 will remain at that level forever. The risk of cardiovascular disease doubles with every increase of 20/10. Remember, everyone with high blood pressure has had a normal reading some time in his or her life! Even if your pressure is normal at age 55, you still have a 90 percent lifetime risk of developing hypertension in the future.

Before starting medications, make whatever lifestyle changes are appropriate in your case. However, give yourself a time limit, such as 2 to 3 months. If your pressure remains high despite your best efforts, start medication while continuing to modify your lifestyle. As you succeed with the latter, you may be able to reduce or eliminate the drugs later on. In the old days, only a few medications were available to treat hypertension, and most of them had adverse effects. Today, there are many more effective and tolerable drugs.

As far as white coat hypertension is concerned, I have a somewhat different take on it than most people. I am impressed by the reports showing that it eventually leads to the same complications as "real" hypertension. I realize that going to a doctor's office can be stressful. I, too, get nervous when someone else takes my pressure. However, isn't life full of stress? If it goes up when your doctor puts the cuff on your arm, won't it also rise when you get your dander up at work, or experience road rage, or feel apprehensive when you hear a police siren behind you when you've been speeding? So many situations in life worry us. The doctor's office is but one. If it happens often enough, regardless of the circumstances, it can undoubtedly strain the vascular system, and should be controlled.

Supermarket Blood Pressure Machines

IF YOU ARE BEING TREATED FOR HIGH BLOOD PRESSURE, or if your pressure is borderline and your doctor is just "watching it," measure it yourself from time to time, away from the doctor's office. It's useful to know your pressure in various situations, and how effectively your medication is working throughout the day.

The best way to monitor your pressure, in my opinion, is with a home blood pressure cuff. Most of these devices are inexpensive, automatic, and easy to use. To make sure the unit is accurate, take it to the doctor's office and check it against the one there.

Many drugstores and supermarkets now have blood pressure machines, providing a convenient, inexpensive, and easy way to measure your blood pressure. You simply slip your arm into a cuff and push a button. But are these machines accurate? Do the stores maintain them, or do they just set them up and forget about them? Frankly, I used to be leery of advising my patients to check their pressure this way, especially in a supermarket.

HERE'S WHAT'S NEW

A nurse in Saskatchewan, Canada, who probably was also dubious of the accuracy of blood pressure measurements in these nonprofessional settings, arranged for four volunteers to test them in 16 randomly selected drugstores and supermarkets throughout the province.

I was happy (and a little surprised) with what she found. Although the recorded readings were a shade high, the last of three consecutive readings taken about a minute apart were apparently reliable.

THE BOTTOM LINE

If you have high blood pressure, check it regularly at your doctor's office. But buy a home unit so you can measure your pressure at home before and after taking medication, eating, or watching an exciting wrestling match—all away from that terrifying white coat! These home kits typically cost less than $100 and usually are reliable. Still, be sure to take yours to your doctor to have its accuracy tested against the professional model.

If you don't have a home unit, it's okay to measure your pressure at the drugstore or supermarket as long as you remember to do it three times. The last reading is the one that counts. If it seems out of line, double-check it at home or with your doctor.

How You Lower Blood Pressure Is Important

LONG-STANDING UNTREATED HIGH BLOOD PRESSURE is a silent killer. It leads to arteriosclerosis (hardening of the arteries) throughout the body, including in the heart, brain, kidney, eyes, and legs. Fortunately, several drugs in different categories can effectively normalize an elevated blood pressure.

Is any one drug better than the others? Until recently, doctors believed that it didn't really matter which medication lowered a patient's pressure as long as the patient tolerated the drug well. Now we know that isn't entirely true. But which drug is best?

HERE'S WHAT'S NEW

The following shows you how important it is to keep up with medical news—almost on a daily basis. In December 2002, the results of a large study carried out in the United States were reported with much fanfare. Researchers followed the clinical course of more than 42,000 people age 55 or older who had hypertension and were being treated with different kinds of blood pressure medication. The purpose of the study was to see whether after 5 years, any one drug that lowers blood pressure more effectively reduced the risk of death, heart attack, or stroke than the others.

Researchers randomly assigned three widely used antihypertensives to the subjects: (1) Hygroton (chlorthalidone), a diuretic or "water pill"; (2) Zestril (lisinopril), an ACE inhibitor; and (3) Norvasc (amlodipine), a calcium channel blocker. To everyone's surprise (including mine), although each drug lowered blood pressure to the same extent, the diuretic resulted in the lowest incidence of heart attack and stroke. Another plus for diuretics is the fact that they cost so much less than the other drugs.

In my opinion, a major shortcoming of this study was the failure to include a beta-blocker, such as Lopressor (metoprolol), or a combined alpha-blocker and beta-blocker, such as Coreg (carvedilol). These drugs are widely prescribed to treat hypertension as well as angina, heart failure, and rhythm disturbances of the heart. It would be important to see how they compare with the diuretics, in light of their many other cardiac benefits.

After this report was made public, I was flooded with phone calls from hypertensive patients who had read these conclusions and who had not been taking a diuretic. They were anxious to switch to the "best" drug, especially considering that diuretics are so much less expensive than the others. I admitted that I was surprised by the findings but happy to make whatever changes were appropriate. However, I cautioned my diabetic patients that diuretics sometimes raise blood glucose levels. I also warned those who had suffered from gout in the past that water pills can elevate uric acid levels in the blood and possibly precipitate an attack of gout. I also reminded them that diuretics are called "water pills" for good reason: They make you "go," something to consider when planning daily activities.

That's where the situation remained for about 2 months, until the next unexpected research bombshell dropped. A large study out of Australia, this one using 6,000 people, found that after 4 years, use of an angiotensin-converting enzyme (ACE) inhibitor resulted in a 17 percent lower incidence of heart attack and stroke *than did a diuretic!*

What was I to tell patients with these two conflicting studies? Fortunately, an even more recent study (in May 2003) resolved my dilemma. This one did not involve a piddling 42,000 subjects like the one that recommended diuretics, or a mere 6,000 like the one that extolled ACE inhibitors. Published in the *Journal of the American Medical Association*, this one reviewed the results of 42 trials embracing 192,478 patients who were followed for an average of 3 to 4 years! The studies compared several combinations of placebo, diuretics, ACE inhibitors, beta-blockers (missing from the first study), calcium-channel blockers, and other blood pressure–lowering agents. They concluded that diuretics are the most effective first-line treatment of high blood pressure for preventing cardiovascular disease.

That settles the matter as far as I am concerned.

THE BOTTOM LINE

Work with your doctor to find the medication or the combination (if more than one drug is necessary) that lowers your blood pressure most effectively with the fewest adverse effects. Try a diuretic first. Most pressures above 160/90 require at least two drugs. The second one should probably be an ACE inhibitor. If you don't tolerate them well (they can cause a dry cough), move on to one of the others, such as an angiotension receptor blocker (ARB) or a beta-blocker.

Lower Your Pressure with Sesame Oil

SESAME OIL is good for you for many reasons. It's rich in mono- and polyunsaturated fatty acids that protect against heart disease and tend to lower cholesterol, and it is also low in dangerous saturated fats. As if that weren't enough, it contains two powerful antioxidants called sesamol and sesamin.

A few years ago, one of my patients developed cancer of the tongue. Usually, by the time this life-threatening malignancy is detected, the tongue has to be removed. Happily, in my patient, the tumor was still very small and localized, permitting treatment with radiation rather than surgery. However, beaming such x-rays toward the sensitive areas of the mouth and throat day after day for weeks leaves the mouth painful and swollen. Swallowing, eating, and talking become very difficult.

Fortunately, this patient had attended one of Dr. Deepak Chopra's seminars in complementary medicine and heard about the use of sesame oil in such cases. She remembered learning that regularly swishing or gargling with sesame oil makes therapeutic radiation of the oral cavity much less unpleasant. She followed this advice and endured a long course of radiation without any ill effect whatsoever. (She subsequently described her experience in a written biography, and some 7 years later she is alive and well.)

I have since learned that the topical application of sesame oil to areas of the skin through which you are receiving radiation also reduces the burning and the irritation caused by such therapy. I have no idea which constituents of sesame oil are responsible for this protection.

HERE'S WHAT'S NEW

As if all these benefits of sesame oil were not enough, researchers have found it has yet another, possibly even more important, action.

It lowers blood pressure! Researchers at India's Annamalai University studied 195 men and 133 women with high blood pressure, all being treated with nifedipine (marketed in this country as Adalat and Procardia). Despite this therapy, the patients' pressures remained above normal. The patients were then asked to do all their cooking with sesame oil while continuing to take the medication. When their blood pressures were measured 60 days later, they were normal in every case.

One can't be sure what components of the sesame oil should be credited with this salutary effect. The study researchers suggest that its mono- and polyunsaturated acids lowered the blood pressure; others credit the antioxidants.

THE BOTTOM LINE

I'm not suggesting that you throw away your blood pressure medication and replace it with sesame oil, especially if it's effective and you're tolerating it. But it seems like a good idea to cook with sesame oil anyway. It has so many other benefits, in addition to being delicious, that you may as well take advantage of its effect on blood pressure.

HIGH CHOLESTEROL

· · · · · · · · · ·

Statins for the Elderly

MIDDLE-AGED MEN AND WOMEN who take statin drugs to reduce their cholesterol levels have fewer heart attacks and lower death rates from coronary artery disease and strokes. But is it too late to take this medication in your seventies and eighties? Some of my older patients think so. "I feel fine. My high cholesterol has never bothered me, so why should I do anything about it at my age? These drugs are expensive and they can cause side effects. Why look for trouble?" Some doctors feel this way too. Are they right?

HERE'S WHAT'S NEW

In a recent study conducted in France, researchers analyzed the results of lowering cholesterol with statin drugs in more than 83,000 patients with coronary artery disease. There were 26 percent fewer strokes when cholesterol levels were kept below 232.

In other research, 20,000 men and women who despite *normal* cholesterol levels had a prior history of heart disease, stroke, and clogged arteries elsewhere in the body, or who had diabetes, were divided into two groups. Half of them received the statin drug Zocor (simvastatin); the others were untreated. Those receiving the Zocor subsequently had one-third fewer recurrent heart attacks or strokes.

In yet another study of almost 6,000 healthy people whose average age was 75 years and who had elevated cholesterol levels, those who took 40 milligrams of Pravachol (pravastatin), for an average of 3.2 years had a 24 percent lower mortality from heart disease than those on a placebo. The incidence of transient ischemic attacks (ministrokes) was also 25 percent less in the treated group.

A study from the Netherlands is reassuring with respect to a possible link between statins and cancer. Comparing the histories of more than 3,000 cancer patients with 16,000 others, those who had taken a statin medication, in this case Zocor, every day for 4 years had a 36 percent *lower* incidence of cancer than those who hadn't. However, the risk of cancer rose to "normal" within 6 months after stopping the statin. So you've got to stay with it.

There seems to be no end to the potential of these statin drugs. We know that they reduce the risk of heart attacks and strokes; they may possibly have an anticancer effect; and now there is evidence that they also protect our brains and bones. In a large study in the United Kingdom, patients 50 years or older on statin therapy were 70 percent less likely to develop Alzheimer's disease than the untreated population. Researchers attribute this benefit to the anti-inflammatory action of the statin drugs.

Another study done in the Netherlands revealed that taking a statin drug for more than a year results in a 36 percent reduction in the incidence of spine fractures. These researchers conclude that the statins prevent bone breakdown and may increase bone density very much as the biphosphonates Fosamax (alendronate) and Actonel (risedronate) do.

THE BOTTOM LINE

I routinely prescribe cholesterol-lowering drugs to every otherwise healthy patient with elevated cholesterol, regardless of age, who has no specific contraindications for its use. Although these drugs are usually well-tolerated, they can sometimes cause muscle, liver, or intestinal problems—side effects that clear up when the drug is discontinued.

In my opinion, if you've had a heart attack or stroke, you should be on a statin drug, regardless of cholesterol level. If you have a family history of heart disease or stroke, discuss with your doctor whether you are a candidate for a statin now, regardless of your cholesterol reading.

INFERTILITY

. . . .

When Miracles Don't Happen

CURRENTLY MORE THAN 5 MILLION AMERICAN COUPLES of child-bearing age want to have a baby and can't. In this country, most women under the age of 30 who engage in regular intercourse will become pregnant within 6 months, but the statistics become less favorable as you grow older.

Infertility is more than a matter of aging would-be moms. Although in every culture it is still widely believed that infertility is strictly a female problem, the truth is that *both* genders contribute equally to the success (or failure) of the reproductive process. Thirty-five percent of infertility cases are due to female hormonal or gynecological problems; another 35 percent are attributable to the male; both partners are responsible in 20 percent of cases; and the cause cannot be determined 10 percent of the time.

Unlike pneumonia, for which you can take an antibiotic, or high blood pressure, which responds to a variety of medications, there is no single treatment for infertility that works for everyone. That's because the problem has many different causes—anatomic, hormonal, or infectious—that must first be identified in both genders.

The most common causes of infertility in women are failure of the ovary to release a mature egg, hormonal deficiencies, endometriosis, previous pelvic infection, vaginal mucus that is hostile to sperm, and structural abnormalities of the genital tract. In men, a decrease in sperm count, a lack of sperm motility, and hormone deficiency are responsible.

Many couples still believe that patience and allowing nature to "take its course" is all that's necessary. However, doctors are now advising couples to seek help sooner rather than later if there is a fertility problem. After 1 year of waiting, there is a 50 percent chance that a specialist can help you. On the other hand, if you keep trying on your own in the hope that you will conceive, the likelihood of having a baby is only 5 percent. If your gynecologist and internist are stumped, consult a fertility specialist if you are younger than 35 and have been trying for 2 years; or if you are between 35 and 40 and have been unsuccessful for 6 months; or if you are over 40 and have had no luck for 3 months. But get such expert help *now* if you have ever had a pelvic infection, a sexually transmitted disease, endometriosis, or gynecological surgery; or if your periods have changed or are irregular, painful, very heavy, or sparse. Also, if you've had two consecutive miscarriages, see a fertility specialist before you try again.

If there is an ovulation problem (determined by ovulation testing), you may need medications to stimulate the ovaries to mature and release an egg. These "fertility pills," usually first taken orally, then by injection if necessary, are powerful hormones that require careful monitoring. Start with Clomid (clomiphene), whose structure is similar to estrogen. It works in a very ingenious way: When it reaches the brain, it attaches itself to the estrogen receptor sites there and blocks them from accepting estrogen. The brain interprets the absence of estrogen in these sites to mean that there is not enough estrogen available and so initiates a series of hormonal changes that increase the production of follicle-stimulating hormone. This causes the ovary to mature its eggs, something that can be determined by ultrasound examination. When one of them is ready, it can, if necessary, be sucked out of the ovary (under local anesthesia in an operating room) to be used for an in vitro fertilization procedure. Clomid is not expensive and is taken orally for 5 days each month. It may cause hot flashes, breast discomfort, and migrainelike headaches. The dose is based on your response.

If your infertility is due to vaginal mucus blocking the entrance to the uterus, your only option may be artificial insemination. In this procedure, sperm is injected directly into the uterus, bypassing the vagina.

If you're a couple beset by infertility, consider these basics:

Try different positions. Everyone relishes the pleasures of making love, but did you know there are optimal positions to increase the chances of a "hit"? If you've had trouble conceiving, you should beg, borrow, or steal a manual that describes the coital positions that favor fertilization.

Check your lubricants. Do not apply a vaginal cream or lubricant that contains a spermicide. Many women are unaware that the nonoxynol-9 they're using for protection against herpes and other infections also kills sperm! Remember, too, that douching after intercourse can affect for sperm.

Keep sperm cool. Sperm don't thrive in high temperatures. That's why men whose testicles have not descended from the abdomen (where they develop) into the cooler environs of the scrotal sac outside the body don't make viable sperm. So if you want to make a baby, don't take a hot bath before intercourse, and don't wear tight shorts that keep the testicles too close to the body, where they are warmed by its higher temperature.

HERE'S WHAT'S NEW

Couples who have had trouble conceiving have heretofore been advised to reduce the frequency of their sexual activity so more sperm can accumulate. That's the wrong thing to do. Recent research indicates that couples should try to have intercourse every 1 to 2 days. Doing so less frequently allows the unused sperm to accumulate and age within the genital areas and lose their potency. Fresh sperm are more likely to fertilize an egg.

In another recent study, Viagra (sildenafil)—of all things—when taken as a vaginal suppository, helped three out of four previously infertile women become pregnant presumably by increasing blood flow to the lining of the uterus, which then enhances the womb's "hospitality" to the fertilized egg.

Taking oral contraceptives for 1 month and then stopping them has been shown to increase the subsequent chances of fertilization! Presumably, they temporarily suppress ovulation, allowing the ovaries to rest so that they can mature their eggs the next time round.

If your infertility problem is causing miscarriages, the following news will be of interest: The length of time between pregnancies is important. Although it seems logical to wait after a stillbirth or miscarriage, that's not the thing to do. According to new research, the longer you delay becoming pregnant again, the greater the risk of stillbirth.

THE BOTTOM LINE

Millions of apparently healthy couples in the United States are infertile. The problem lies equally with the man and the woman, and sometimes both contribute to it. In some 10 percent of cases, the cause of the infertility remains an enigma.

Consult your doctor about getting the necessary tests to discover the reason for your infertility. Researchers have discovered some promising new techniques to help correct it. If none of these help, there are powerful in vitro fertilization tools with a high rate of success that involve mating selected sperm and egg in a laboratory dish and implanting the fertilized egg into the uterus.

IRREGULAR HEARTBEAT (ATRIAL FIBRILLATION)

* * * * * * * * *

Another Cause and a New Approach

MANY OF US have a slightly irregular cardiac rhythm from time to time, usually a harmless "extra beat"—something that does not require treatment. Atrial fibrillation (AF), on the other hand, is the most common *significant* cardiac rhythm disturbance in this country. It affects about 2.2 million people in the United States, and 160,000 new cases are reported every year. (Don't confuse *atrial* fibrillation with *ventricular* fibrillation (VF), however. AF is common and manageable; VF, on the other hand, results in almost instantaneous loss of consciousness and ends in death if it continues for longer than 4 to 6 minutes.)

Atrial fibrillation manifests itself as a persistent and totally irregular heartbeat. It can occur now and then interspersed with long intervals of normal heart rhythm, but in many cases it is permanent. Although patients usually can tell whether they're "fibrillating" (they perceive it as an irregular pounding sometimes accompanied by shortness of breath, chest discomfort, or both), many are unaware of it and it is detected during a routine physical.

The atria are small chambers sitting atop each of the much larger ventricles. The atria normally send impulses to the ventricles (the pump of the heart) causing them to contract. The atria generate 60 to 80 such impulses per minute in a regular rhythm. In patients with AF, these impulses are disorganized, chaotic, and occur 300 to 600 times a minute. Fortunately, not all of them "get through." If the ventricles had to respond to everyone of these stimuli, they would soon be exhausted. However, as many as 170 or even 180 impulses can reach the ventricles every minute, forcing them to contract in a rapid, haphazard way. This fast, irregular beating is what creates the symptoms that many patients with this disorder experience.

Every case of AF must be thoroughly evaluated to determine what caused it—and it must be treated. The arrhythmia itself, when correctly managed, is not a threat to life or its quality. Most cases of AF stem from some other underlying "condition," such as coronary artery disease, untreated high blood pressure, one or more abnormally functioning cardiac valves (especially the mitral), heart failure, chronic lung disease, a traveling blood clot to the lungs (pulmonary embolus), disease of the heart muscle (cardiomyopathy), inflammation of the thin envelope that surrounds the heart (pericarditis), or congenital heart disease. An overactive thyroid gland can also cause AF. A recent alcoholic binge can do it, as can too much caffeine, serious stress, use of stimulant drugs or decongestants, severe infection, or an imbalance of body chemicals due to medications such as diuretics. The significance and long-term outlook for someone with AF depends a great deal on its underlying cause. For example, if it's due to excessive use of some drug, it should never recur. However, if it's associated with a diseased mitral heart valve, it's apt to be permanent.

In about 10 percent of cases, AF develops in the absence of any discernible disease, cardiac or otherwise. Some years ago, it was detected during a routine exam in a perfectly healthy astronaut training to go to the moon. It began at age 54 in one of my patients who continued to lead a normal, active life as a United States senator until he died of "natural" causes at age 86.

After establishing the cause of your AF, your doctor will usually try to restore normal heart rhythm. Although there are several medications that can do so, including some new ones, they don't always work. If they fail, your doctor may then try to convert the AF to normal rhythm by means of electroshock, which can be done on an outpatient basis. You are given short-acting sedative or anesthetic that knocks you out for a couple of minutes. Paddles are placed on your chest, and a current is delivered to the heart through the chest wall. You feel nothing and, in many cases, you awake to a normal rhythm. It's often successful.

If normal cardiac rhythm cannot be restored by drugs or maintained after electroshock, your doctor should start you on a medication to control the rate at which the ventricles beat. The goal should be between 60 and 80 beats per minute, which can be achieved by various drugs including beta-blockers, calcium channel blockers, and digitalis.

You should also be started on a blood thinner such as Coumadin (warfarin), because the greatest danger of AF is a stroke. That's because even when you control the rate at which the ventricles beat, the atria continue to beat very rapidly. As a result, they don't contract completely. Instead of blood being expelled into the ventricles on its way to the rest of the body, it just stagnates. This permits clots to form that can then enter the ventricles that squeeze them out into circulation to the brain. If you don't tolerate the warfarin well, aspirin is the next best substitute.

If the heart rate cannot be kept within a reasonable range or the AF continues to make you uncomfortable, you may be a candidate for an invasive ablation procedure. ("Ablation" is defined as the removal of diseased or unwanted tissue from the body by surgical or other means. In this case, it's with electrical energy, not surgery.) There are two types of ablation procedure. In one, a catheter threaded up to your heart from a vein in the groin delivers high-frequency electrical energy that destroys or inactivates the area in the atria from which the abnormal impulses originate. This leaves the heart fibrillating, but slowly. So slowly, in fact, that you may sometimes need a pacemaker to keep it going fast enough.

The other ablation procedure blocks impulses originating in a pulmonary vein through which blood normally flows back from the heart to the lungs for reoxygenation. This ablation procedure is somewhat more difficult to do and carries with it a risk of clots forming in the treated vein. However, when it is successful (70 to 80 percent of cases), the AF is converted to normal rhythm. If you decide to go this route, make sure the procedure is done at a hospital that has a good track record with it.

HERE'S WHAT'S NEW

Sleep apnea has been recently identified as yet another contributing factor of AF—and a treatable one at that. A study at the Mayo Clinic found that people with untreated sleep apnea are twice as likely to develop AF as are those with normal sleep patterns. When sleep apnea in patients with AF was left untreated, the arrhythmia recurred in more than 80 percent of them. When the apnea was eliminated, the AF returned in only 42 percent. Sleep apnea is treated with continuous positive air pressure that keeps the airways open during the night (see page 148).

Doctors are taking a new approach to treating AF. Many now believe that it's less important to restore normal rhythm than it is to keep the heart beating at an acceptable rate and to prevent clots from forming and traveling to the brain. The fact is you can live quite normally with AF if the latter two conditions are met. So don't worry if your doctor is unable to "break" the AF. Just make sure to take your anticoagulant and that your medication keeps your heart rate under 80 beats per minute.

THE BOTTOM LINE

If you've developed AF, consider sleep apnea as a possible cause in addition to the others described above. Normalizing your nighttime breathing may abolish your cardiac arrhythmia or make it easier to control.

Although there are many ways to restore normal rhythm in someone with AF, they are not always successful. However, remember that you can have AF and still live a virtually normal life. More important than trying to keep your heart rhythm normal is to make sure that it is not beating too fast, and that you take a blood thinner for as long as the fibrillation persists. And that may be a lifetime.

WHAT THE DOCTOR ORDERED?

NEW HOME TEST FOR CHECKING BLOOD THINNER DOSAGE ● Millions of Americans who take an anticoagulant (blood thinner), such as Coumadin (warfarin), also need to monitor their blood regularly. They require this medication for several possible reasons:

- They have atrial fibrillation, a common irregular cardiac rhythm in which blood clots can form in the heart, travel to the brain, and result in a stroke.

- They have had a stroke (due to a hemorrhage or clogged artery in the brain) or heart attack and require "blood thinning" to prevent a recurrence.

- They have one or more blood clots in the veins of the legs that may or may not have already traveled to the lungs (pulmonary embolism).

- They have a mechanical heart valve.

- They suffer from a blood clotting disorder.

Anticoagulants prevent the formation of blood clots, stop their spread, or both. However, these anticoagulants are not without risk. Unless their dose is carefully monitored at frequent and regular intervals, the blood can become too "thin" and result in bleeding or hemorrhage anywhere in the body, especially in the bowel and brain, or is not "thin" enough, placing them at risk for stroke or pulmonary embolism.

To prevent these complications, patients must have their blood analyzed every 3 to 4 weeks. This means going to a clinic or the doctor's office and waiting for the results later that day, at which time your dosage is adjusted until the next test in 3 to 4 weeks. This is time-consuming, expensive, and inconvenient, and especially difficult for people who travel. It isn't always easy to find a facility where the test is done accurately and where results are available before your plane leaves.

HERE'S WHAT'S NEW • LifeScan, a Johnson & Johnson company, has developed the Harmony INR Monitoring System, a do-it-yourself device that patients can use at home to determine their international normalized ratio (INR), the standard measurement of blood clotting time. It's cheaper and more convenient than having it done at a laboratory, and most important, you get the results immediately. Telephone them to the doctor, and receive your medication instructions there and then. The great advantage of this device is that you can check your coagulation status as often as you want, preferably weekly instead of monthly. This should cut down on complications that result from blood that is too thin or not thin enough.

You can buy your own Harmony monitor with a prescription. It's easy to use. You prick your finger, place a drop of blood onto a test strip, insert it (the strip, not the finger) into the monitor, and presto, in 90 seconds you have your answer!

THE BOTTOM LINE • There's no downside to the Harmony monitor. Ask your doctor about it. It's easy to use, less expensive, and very much more convenient. •

IRRITABLE BOWEL
SYNDROME

· · · · · · · · ·

Communication Breakdown

SOME 10 MILLION TO 20 MILLION American adults have a "nervous stomach," or are plagued by chronic "indigestion" or "heartburn," nausea and vomiting, bloating, stomach distension with frequent belching, flatulence, constipation and/or diarrhea, and the feeling that there's something left after a bowel movement. Their stool often consists of long, ropy strands with mucus. These symptoms, and nature's perennial calls to "go" or "fart" frequently and unpredictably, leave millions of us focused on our guts—and always needing to know the location of the nearest toilet, just in case.

Doctors have a variety of names for this condition: *irritable bowel syndrome (IBS), functional GI (short for gastrointestinal) disorder, spastic colon*, and *mucus colitis*. Whatever you call it (I prefer IBS), this disorder is responsible for almost half of all visits to doctors' offices because of digestive complaints. It is probably the second most frequent cause of absenteeism from work (after the common cold).

Doctors are now able to recognize, diagnose, and treat IBS more effectively than ever. Traditionally, such patients would wander from doctor to doctor looking for an answer and a cure. They'd get neither. Instead they would endure repeated colonoscopies, stool analyses, barium x-rays, CT scans, and MRIs of the abdomen—all of which would invariably come up "normal." Despite this "clean bill of health," they'd continue to ache, cramp, fart, and run to the john all day. The reassurance that their misery was "nothing serious" or life-threatening was small comfort.

It's frequently agreed that IBS is the result of a breakdown in the normal communication between the brain and the bowel. The chronic belly pain, spasm, constipation, and diarrhea develop because the nerves supplying the gut are either hypersensitive or sluggish. When they send fewer signals to the bowel, the stool passes more slowly down the intestinal tract and the result is constipation; when the nervous activity is excessive, the stools are frequent and liquid.

No one knows why some people have IBS and others don't, or why it fluctuates in severity. It sometimes follows a stressful event, such as divorce, bereavement, or simply a poor report card. However, symptoms usually continue long after the event that it provoked and forgotten. Chronic stress does not cause IBS, but it can worsen its symptoms. Although there is no cure for IBS, the quality of life for those who suffer from it can be improved.

If your symptoms suggest IBS, make sure that they are not due to something else. Ask for a comprehensive workup to exclude a host of curable conditions that produce a similar clinical picture. The necessary tests include a complete blood count, liver profile, stool analyses, CT scan of the abdomen, and a colonoscopy or flexible sigmoidoscopy.

The following conditions mimic irritable bowel syndrome:

Lactose intolerance. Most of us make too little lactase, the enzyme that digests lactose (the sugar present in milk and milk products). Undigested lactose in the gut can imitate some of the symptoms of IBS, the severity of which depends on the degree of its deficiency.

Medication. Every medication you're taking, whether it's a vitamin, supplement, or herb, is suspect when you have any chronic bowel complaint. If you have symptoms of IBS, discontinue every medication that is not absolutely necessary. I've often cured diarrhea simply by eliminating excessive doses of various vitamins.

Infection. People with the symptoms of IBS often turn out to have unrecognized bacterial, fungal, or parasitic infection. When the infection—be it an amoeba, giardia, or *Clostridium difficile*—is eradicated, the stomach stops being "nervous."

Malabsorption. When the pancreas doesn't make enough of its enzymes, food remains undigested in the intestinal tract and can cause symptoms identical to those of IBS. The presence of these enzymes is simple to determine, and, if lacking, they are easy to replace.

Food allergies or sensitivities. These account for a surprising number of chronic bowel symptoms. Any food, no matter how bland or "good" it is for you, can make you sick if you're allergic to it. Skin testing as well as elimination diets can identify the culprit food.

Sprue or celiac disease. Patients with this common disorder who eat wheat, barley, and rye to which they are allergic, develop bloating, gas, diarrhea, and constipation.

Inflammatory bowel disease (IBD). This disease (Crohn's or ulcerative colitis) can mimic irritable bowel syndrome, but the treatment and outlook are very different.

HERE'S WHAT'S NEW

Here's what to do after all the other possibilities have been ruled out and you are left with the diagnosis of IBS.

Modify your diet. Avoid any food that causes or worsens your symptoms. Limit your intake of milk and milk products in case your IBS is a result of lactose deficiency. Eat plenty of fiber and little fat. Wheat bran, oat bran, barley, peas, and a variety of vegetables are all fiber-rich. You can also add fiber supplements to your diet. My favorite ones are FiberCon, Prodiem, and Fibermed. If you have diarrhea, avoid tomatoes and strawberries.

Follow a bowel routine. Go to the bathroom at the same time every day, preferably after a meal, and give yourself enough time to finish the job.

Apply heat. A heating pad or a hot bath may provide relief from abdominal cramps or pain.

Reduce stress. Even though stress and emotional distress are not the prime causes of IBS, they can worsen symptoms. Ask your doctor about biofeedback, hypnosis, and relaxation therapy, all of which can be useful.

Stay active. Exercise for at least 20 minutes every day.

If you smoke, stop!

Try medication. Imodium, Lomotil, and Pepto-Bismol control diarrhea. Abdominal cramps are eased by antispasmodic drugs such as Levsin (hyoscyamine), Librax (chloramphenicol), or Bentyl (dicyclomine).

Avoid stimulant laxatives. If you're chronically constipated, use osmotic laxatives, such as sorbitol or lactulose, which draw water into the bowel and make it easier to eliminate stool.

THE BOTTOM LINE

IBS is a chronic disorder that begins in young adult life and usually becomes less severe as you age. It is characterized by irritability of the colon that fluctuates between diarrhea and constipation. There's no known cause, and a complete gastrointestinal workup fails to reveal any structural, physical, or chemical abnormalities. Despite the troublesome and often embarrassing symptoms, IBS does not lead to cancer and does not shorten life. There is no cure or specific treatment, but you'll feel better if you keep your bowels regular, eat a high-fiber diet, and take antispasmodic drugs when needed. Do not accept a diagnosis of IBS before your gastrointestinal tract has been thoroughly evaluated.

KIDNEY STONES

• • • • • • • • • •

Curb the Real Culprit

AT LEAST ONE MILLION AMERICANS, most of them between ages 20 and 40, suffer a kidney stone attack every year. Overall, there is a 1 in 10 chance that you will develop and pass such a stone sometime during your life. And that likelihood is even greater if you are a woman or have a close family member with kidney stones.

A kidney stone attack has been called "worse than childbirth" (not that the men making these assertions would know!), and have afflicted humankind for thousands of years. Although stones can strike anyone, some people are more vulnerable than others.

Normally, the various substances present in urine are in balance with one another and remain dissolved. People who make kidney stones lack certain chemical "inhibitors" in the urine that prevent its constituents from solidifying.

Here is what having a kidney stone feels like:

- Pain, often sharp and coming in waves, begins suddenly in the back and the side where the kidneys are located. As the stone makes its may along the urinary ducts, the pain radiates toward the groin. It may ease up temporarily when the stone stops, but it recurs once it starts moving again.

- Blood in the urine, visible under the microscope if not to the naked eye. Urine is also apt to be cloudy or foul-smelling when there is infection in the urinary tract.

- Nausea and vomiting.

- Fever, chills, and weakness, especially when infection is present.

- Urinary frequency and urgency when the stone reaches the very end of the ureter (the tube that carries urine from the kidney to the bladder).

Prevention and treatment depend on the composition of the stone. So it's important to "catch" any stone you pass and have it analyzed. The most common kidney stone consists of calcium oxalate. Other types are ones composed of uric acid (in people with gout who have high uric acid levels) or struvite (found in those with chronic infection of the kidneys). The rest are caused by a few rare metabolic and genetic disorders.

Your doctor should perform a CT scan of the abdomen to confirm the presence of a stone to determine its size and location. If the stone doesn't pass by itself (most do), there are several ways to remove it by minimally invasive treatments.

HERE'S WHAT'S NEW

Since almost 95 percent of kidney stones contain some calcium, doctors used to advise patients with these stones to reduce the calcium in their diets. Women who needed calcium to prevent osteoporosis were in a quandary. Should they take it and run the risk of kidney stones, or avoid it and suffer fractures from osteoporosis? Happily, research has shown that *oxalate*—not calcium—is the real villain. Avoiding calcium-rich foods can actually result in *more* stone formation, but don't take calcium oxalate tablets and calcium-rich antacids. The combination of calcium and oxalate is what makes these stones; calcium alone doesn't do it. So reduce your intake of oxalate and maintain or *increase* your consumption of dietary calcium. You won't be able to eliminate all the oxalate from your diet, but you can cut back by not eating foods that are richest in it such as beets, collard greens, dry cocoa, spinach, and turnip greens.

Another trend I expect will have an impact on the formation of kidney stones is the bottled water boom. The most important factor in kidney stone formation is dehydration, usually the result of not drinking enough water. This is most likely to happen when you're perspiring excessively in hot weather and exercising vigorously. When you're dehydrated, the constituents of urine, especially mineral salts such as calcium, tend to come out of solution and form tiny crystals.

People everywhere these days are swigging from disposable plastic water bottles—on the streets, in subways and on buses, in classrooms, arenas, football games, baseball games, board meetings, and doctors' waiting rooms. Bottled water breaks have replaced the smoke break! Even though the incidence of kidney stones has been increasing in the past two decades, the next count may well show a reversal of that trend because of this fad (of which I approve).

THE BOTTOM LINE

Doctors used to tell their patients with kidney stones to reduce their calcium intake. This is unnecessary, and in fact may lead to more stones. The major offender is the oxalate in foods. Another key to the prevention and treatment of all kidney stones is drinking enough water to produce at least 2 quarts of urine a day.

LUPUS

* * * * * * * * *

A New Treatment

THE NORMAL IMMUNE SYSTEM has "killer cells" that attack and destroy harmful bacteria, cancer cells, and other threats to the body. In a group of diseases called autoimmune disorders, the immune system malfunctions and these killer cells attack and destroy healthy tissue instead of harmful "invaders." One such disease, lupus, afflicts almost 1.5 million Americans, mostly women.

Lupus strikes various organs randomly and unpredictably—the joints, heart, lungs, kidney, liver, and the vascular system. Conventional treatment, not always successful, consists of drugs that suppress the immune system and prevent the killer cells from continuing to go awry. The most widely used of these medications are the cytotoxic anticancer drugs. They usually are given in small monthly doses that gradually eliminate the malfunctioning immune cells. However, these agents ultimately destroy the bone marrow, so doctors traditionally remove some of the patient's marrow cells beforehand and return them after the treatment is completed to "repopulate" the marrow. This regimen sometimes works, but the results are nothing to write home about and improvement doesn't usually last long. Most patients remain chronically sick.

HERE'S WHAT'S NEW

Doctors at the Johns Hopkins Medical Center in Baltimore have been trying a new approach. Instead of a slow, gradual attack on the immune system, they swiftly wipe out the rogue cells with high doses of Cytoxan (cyclophosphamide), a cytotoxic chemotherapy drug. And they no longer remove bone marrow for reinjection later because it may be diseased and make the patient sick again. Although cyclophosphamide destroys the bone marrow, the doctors have found that the immature stem cells normally present in it are unaffected by the drug and free from disease. When treatment is stopped, they take over and produce normal marrow.

The Hopkins group has tried this therapy on only 14 patients, but researchers are optimistic about the results. About 2½ years later, five patients were completely free from disease, and six had improved enough to tolerate and respond to a drug that had not worked before; only three had little or no benefit.

THE BOTTOM LINE

These results are so impressive that three more major medical centers have started clinical trials with this therapy. I'm reporting this news so that if you, or someone you know, has lupus and are not doing well, you will contact one of these institutions and find out about participating in their study. The centers are: Drexel University College of Medicine in Philadelphia, the Medical College of Wisconsin, and Johns Hopkins Medical Center. You can also call the Lupus Center at (410) 614-1573 for more information or e-mail them at stdman@jhmi.edu.

LYME DISEASE

. . . .

Don't Overtreat It

LYME DISEASE IS CAUSED BY A BACTERIUM called *Borrelia burgdorferi*. You become infected when you are bitten by a tick that has fed on an animal (typically a white-tailed deer) that happens to be harboring this bug. Most of the 16,000 new cases of Lyme disease each year in the United States occur in spring when the tick is in the nymph stage (very tiny) and less likely to be seen than in fall when it is in the larval stage and bigger.

More than half of patients with Lyme disease don't know they've been bitten and first suspect the disease when they develop the signature bull's-eye rash. This is sometimes accompanied by flulike symptoms. The rash usually persists for 2 to 4 weeks. This early stage of the disease is the best time to treat it. However, the disease may not be easy to recognize in patients who sometimes never develop the rash. If the diagnosis is missed early on, the infection can involve the joints, the heart, and the brain, resulting in disabling, chronic disease.

The three most widely used antibiotics to treat Lyme disease are Vibramycin (doxycycline), Augmentin (amoxicillin), and Ceftin (cefuroxime). The prescribed drug is taken orally for 3 to 4 weeks.

HERE'S WHAT'S NEW

A team of researchers led by Gary Wormser, M.D., a recognized authority in this disease at New York Medical College, studied 180 Lyme disease patients. All of them followed one of three antibiotic dosage schedules after the appearance of the rash: (1) 20 days of doxycycline, (2) 10 days of doxycycline, or (3) 10 days of doxycycline and one intravenous dose of Rocephin (ceftriaxone), another antibiotic.

When the patients were reevaluated 3 months later, Dr. Wormser found that 85 to 90 percent of them had completely recovered regardless of which antibiotic treatment they received. In other words, continuing the doxycycline for 20 days rather than 10, or adding the second antibiotic conferred no additional benefit. In fact, it was likely to result in a greater incidence of adverse effects such as diarrhea.

According to Dr. Wormser, "Shorter courses of treatment are safer, less expensive, and may be less likely to promote emergence of resistant bacteria that can endanger the entire community." The widespread unnecessary use of antibiotics or higher-than-required doses for too long a time may result in the emergence of bacteria that are resistant to them. Several such strains of bacteria have already appeared and are causing serious, even life-threatening, infections.

THE BOTTOM LINE

If you live in tick country (especially rural areas of the northeast United States, Wisconsin, Minnesota, or Northern California) consider Lyme disease if you're tired, achy, have frequent headaches, and generally feel out of sorts for no apparent reason. You may have missed the rash caused by a tick bite. Regardless of whether or not you see one, let your doctor know how you feel. (The average person with Lyme disease consults as many as five doctors before the correct diagnosis is made.)

If you are diagnosed with Lyme disease in its early stages, you need a much shorter course of antibiotics than has been traditionally given. If more prolonged therapy is recommended, refer your doctor to the paper published in the *Annals of Internal Medicine*, Volume 138, as well as the accompanying supporting editorial by Allen Steere, M.D., who unraveled the disease in Lyme, Connecticut, nearly 30 years ago.

MENOPAUSE

· · · · · · · · ·

Questioning Hormone Replacement Therapy

GIVEN THE EVER-INCREASING LIFE SPAN in the United States, an American woman can expect to be menopausal for about one-third of her life. Little wonder there is so much research, discussion, and debate about the treatment of this "condition."

At the root of menopause are hormonal changes. When women reach their forties, they begin to make less estrogen, the main female hormone. Its production decreases gradually for several years, during which time periods become irregular and insomnia, fatigue, mood swings, and hot flashes develop. The period during which estrogen production wanes is called perimenopause. Then, sometime between ages 48 and 55, and in 1 percent of those under 40, the periods stop. One year after your last one, you are officially menopausal.

How you feel while all this is happening, and indeed during the rest of your life, is unpredictable. Some women remain troubled by the signature symptoms of menopause—the hot flashes and flushes, night sweats, depression, irritability, vaginal dryness, and loss of libido. Others barely notice them. Regardless of how you feel, things are happening of which you won't be aware until later because lack of estrogen affects organs everywhere in the body. You may be developing osteoporosis with brittle bones that break easily; arteries may be hardening and narrowing (arteriosclerosis), leaving you vulnerable to a heart attack or stroke. Replacement of this hormone was traditionally the treatment of choice to minimize symptoms and minimize future problems.

HERE'S WHAT'S NEW

Most recently, virtually everything that was supposed to be good about replacing estrogen has been refuted. Mind you, there were always two schools of thought about hormone replacement therapy (HRT). The first (and less vocal) always maintained that nature must know what it's doing when it has the ovaries stop making these hormones. They advised against taking hormone replacements and tampering with this normal course of events. If nature had wanted women to continue to have estrogen later in life, the argument went, it would have designed the female body to keep producing it.

The HRT proponents scoffed at this simplistic reasoning. They argued that nature makes lots of mistakes (such as allowing cells to grow wildly and cause cancer) and that menopause is one of them. This natural error, they claimed, is why humans are one of the only mammals that have a menopause. They were adamant that it should be replaced.

Over the years, there were scores of studies (most of which, in retrospect, appear to have been flawed) "proving" that HRT protects menopausal woman from a host of ailments. HRT proponents pointed out that it controls hot flashes, mood swings, dry vaginal tissue, aging skin, and brittle bones and also reduces the risk of heart disease, stroke, and Alzheimer's disease. These doctors (I was one of them) admitted that estrogen can cause cancer of the uterus, but that could be prevented by adding progesterone. Breast cancer? We were not convinced by the data available at the time, they said, and anyway, if every woman had an annual mammogram, it would detect these cancers early enough to cure them. All in all, the estrogen school of thought made HRT look logical—and the evidence supporting its many benefits seemed incontrovertible. More important, millions of women who took these hormone supplements looked and felt better.

Then came the statisticians and the epidemiologists. One by one, they disproved virtually every claim about estrogen. They showed that this hormone doesn't protect against heart attack and stroke and, in fact, actually causes them! Doubts that estrogen contributes to breast cancer also disappeared. Estrogen's few confirmed benefits, such as reducing the severity of osteoporosis and controlling night sweats and hot flashes, were overshadowed by its many dangers.

One remaining myth that estrogen improves memory and slows progression of Alzheimer's was refuted in a large double-blind, randomized, placebo-controlled study in 39 clinical centers throughout the United States. The purpose of this research was to assess the effect of HRT on the incidence of dementia and cognitive impairment in women ages 65 and older. Of the 4,500 women in the trial, about half received the standard estrogen-progestin combination; the other half was given a placebo. Women who took the hormones for an average of slightly more than 4 years actually had twice the incidence of Alzheimer's or other forms of dementia compared with those taking a placebo! This increase translates into only 23 more cases among every 10,000 women taking the hormone. It doesn't sound like much—unless you happen to be one of them! The HRT did not protect against mild memory loss either.

Another study of 16,000 women ages 50 to 79, followed for an average of 5.6 years, was stopped 3 years early because those receiving HRT had a 44 percent *increased* risk of stroke compared with those on placebo.

THE BOTTOM LINE

These studies did not involve women under 65, and in all cases, the estrogen was being taken along with progestin. Subsequent research has yielded similar results when estrogen was taken alone. All these data constitute a strong case against using these hormones for most women. This conclusion is further strengthened by the findings in the government-supported Women's Health Initiative that women taking hormones are at higher risk for heart attack, stroke, and breast cancer.

Are there any safe alternatives to help control some of the troubling symptoms of estrogen deprivation? If you are experiencing hot flashes and night sweats, try one of the newer selective serotonin reuptake inhibitors (SSRIs), such as the antidepressant Paxil (paroxetine). However, do so under close medical supervision.

Some doctors recommend that women consume natural soy products (such as tofu or soy milk) to help minimize the symptoms of menopause. Asian women have a much lower incidence of hot flashes, as well as fewer estrogen-dependent tumors such as breast cancer. It is widely believed that's because instead of taking estrogen supplements, these women follow a diet rich in phytoestrogens, which are weaker natural estrogen-like hormones. When the body stops making estrogen and the estrogen receptors to which this hormone is bound are empty (resulting in all of the typical menopausal symptoms), these phytoestrogens take over. They bind to the estrogen receptors, where they act as weaker versions of the hormone.

The phytoestrogens with the greatest estrogen effects are genistein and daidzein, both present in soya and its compounds. Some women who take soy supplements have fewer hot flashes and may be less likely to develop osteoporosis than those who are not on any hormonal supplements. However, the overall benefit remains uncertain and undocumented. Soybeans contain all eight essential fatty acids and so are a better source of protein than is milk, yet do not have the latter's fat or cholesterol. Several other plant phytoestrogens are also sold in health food stores. Among them are dong quai (Chinese angelica), wild yams, black cohosh, and milk thistle.

If none of the soy products help and only estrogen seems to work, take the lowest effective HRT dose for the shortest possible time. If you have vaginal problems such as dryness or irritation, use the topical estrogen creams. They appear to be safe. For the prevention and treatment of osteoporosis, there are many new drugs that work at least as well as estrogen (see pages 248 and 269).

Evista Benefits

WOMEN WHO HAVE GONE THROUGH MENOPAUSE are at increased risk for bone loss because they are no longer protected by estrogen. What should women now take to prevent bone loss?

The drug Evista (raloxifene) is a selective estrogen receptor modulator widely used to prevent and treat osteoporosis. Although it's neither estrogen nor even a hormone, it does have some estrogen-like properties, the most important of which is its ability to reduce bone loss and increase bone density (thus preventing and/or minimizing osteoporosis). It does not adversely affect the breast and uterus the way estrogen does, so it does not cause cancer of those organs, tenderness of the breast, or vaginal bleeding. On the other hand it does not relieve symptoms of menopause, such as hot flashes, either.

HERE'S WHAT'S NEW

Data from a 4-year study of almost 8,000 postmenopausal women revealed that a subset of about 1,000 women with one or more risk factors for cardiovascular disease who were taking Evista to control osteoporosis had a 40 percent lower risk of developing heart disease and a 62 percent reduction in the risk of all fatal and nonfatal strokes. (They also enjoyed a 70 percent decline in the incidence of breast cancer.)

THE BOTTOM LINE

Evista has a beneficial effect on heart disease, stroke, and breast cancer with few side effects other than a small increased risk of clot formation in the veins. For that reason, anyone with varicose veins or a history of thrombophlebitis should not use it, nor should those women who are premenopausal or pregnant. However, in my opinion, virtually every postmenopausal female at risk for osteoporosis—especially those also vulnerable to heart disease, stroke, and breast cancer—should take it.

MIGRAINE

● ● ● ● ● ● ● ● ● ●

Keep Your Head Together

ASK ANYONE WHO'S HAD THEM, migraines are not just ordinary headaches—they are all-consuming. A migraine headache won't kill you, but when you're in its throes, you may wish it would.

Migraine often starts with a warning sign or "prodrome." You suddenly feel very tired, you have no appetite, your mood changes for no apparent reason, and you become sensitive to bright light or loud sounds. You may see an "aura" of flashing lights, zigzag lines, stars or shimmery sheets; your vision becomes blurred; there are blind spots before you; or you develop tunnel vision (you can see only what's straight ahead and not on either side). You may be unable to speak clearly and you may feel confused, an arm or leg may be weak, your face may tingle or feel numb. Minutes, hours, or even a day or two later, the headache itself strikes—an all-consuming, severe throbbing, pounding, blinding pain on one side of your head—around the eye, the forehead, ear, jaw, and temple. As if this weren't enough, you are also nauseated and may even vomit. Some patients develop diarrhea or increased urination. Light and loud noises are unbearable; you feel cold and you look pale. All this agony lasts from a few hours to several days.

More people than ever are suffering from migraine. Its incidence has increased 60 percent in the past 10 years so that one American in 10 is now a "migraineur." It can occur at any age and affects three times as many women (most of them premenopausal) as men. Children, too, have migraine, but in them it produces recurrent cyclical vomiting rather than headache.

Migraine is such a miserable disorder and affects so many people that doctors and researchers are working very hard to find ways to control it. We've come a long way in treating migraine since the Stone Age when the only therapy was to cut away a piece of the skull in order to liberate the "evil spirits."

Despite intense research for many years, the cause of migraine remains unclear. Until quite recently, it was believed to be purely vascular in origin—narrowing of the arteries in the head followed by their dilation. However, newer imaging techniques and a better understanding of the chemical changes within the brain suggest that migraine is a disorder of the brain rather than its blood vessels. Changes in blood flow, though important, are secondary. Some process inside the brain is believed to trigger the migraine attack by altering the concentration of some of its chemicals—the neurotransmitters serotonin, norepinephrine, and dopamine—this, in turn, leads to the release of pain-causing substances.

Other researchers believe that a migraine "generator" in the brain stimulates the nerves to constrict the blood vessels in the face, scalp, spinal cord, and the membranes covering the brain. This decreases the amount of oxygen available to the brain, and accounts for the difficulty with speech, confusion, and visual changes. In order to restore the blood supply, other arteries in the brain dilate, causing the release of pain-producing substances called prostaglandins. The dilated arteries and prostaglandins responsible for the blinding migraine headache. Since the brain itself does not sense pain, the pain is felt in the tissues covering it, as well as in the muscles and blood vessels around the scalp, face, and neck.

There are many "triggers": straining at stool, fasting, low blood sugar, high altitudes, a falling barometer, a sudden change in temperature, fatigue, glaring or flickering lights, or motion sickness. Ingredients in more than 100 foods can also do so. These include the tyramine and phenylethylamine in cheese, meat, seafood, peas, pickles, olives, sauerkraut, and various alcoholic beverages (look for them on every food label); the tannin in apple juice, coffee, red wine, and tea; the sulfites in wine; the monosodium glutamate in Chinese food; various other chemicals in chocolate, yogurt, and nuts. In half of all female sufferers migraine comes on during the first three days of their period.

Tried-and-true measures remain your best bet for treating a migraine attack. To relieve the pain, start with the least potent medications. A good over-the-counter drug to try first is Excedrin Extra Strength (a combination of acetaminophen, aspirin, and caffeine). A nonsteroidal anti-inflammatory drug (NSAID) such as Advil (ibuprofen) or Aleve (naproxen) is equally effective first-line therapy. Remember that high doses of these agents can irritate the stomach lining, so look out for belly pain and black stools (evidence of intestinal bleeding). Since migraine is a chronic problem, use narcotic medications only as a last resort lest you end up dependent on them.

The triptans are a major advance in the treatment of migraine. First there was Imitrex (sumatriptan), followed by a number of related preparations, including Zomig (zolmitriptan), Amerge (naratriptan), Maxalt (rizatriptan), and several others. They are prescription drugs that work by increasing serotonin levels in the brain that narrow the dilated, pulsating arteries. They take effect quickly, especially the newer ones, and should be used at the very onset of symptoms. Triptans come in several forms: pills, wafers that dissolve under the tongue, injections, and nasal sprays. However, since they constrict the blood vessels, they can also cause stroke and heart attack in people with arteriosclerosis, vascular disease, high blood pressure, coronary artery disease, or poorly controlled diabetes. Avoid them if you have any of these problems. They should also be avoided by anyone with severe asthma. Selective serotonin uptake inhibitors (SSRIs), antidepressants whose prototype is Prozac (fluoxetine), also increase serotonin, so don't use them along with the triptans. Pregnant women should not take triptans because their effect on the fetus has not been determined.

The various triptans differ in their terms of adverse effects and duration of action. Frova (frovatriptan), the latest one approved by the FDA, is said to have fewer side effects and remains in the blood for about 26 hours longer than any of the others.

Another drug to consider is dihydroergotamine (DHE). It's available as a nasal spray. I sometimes prescribe it for patients in whom other treatments provide only temporary relief.

Prevention is as important in migraine as it is for any other disease. If you are a "migraineur," try to:

Eat right and stay active. Follow a diet low in fat and rich in complex carbohydrates. Exercise regularly, and when you do, warm up gradually because sudden aerobic exercise can precipitate the headaches.

Try mind over matter. Mind-body techniques, biofeedback, yoga, transcutaneous electrical nerve stimulation, and tai chi all help by reducing stress.

Beware of hormones. Avoid oral contraceptives, especially if you smoke or have a family history of stroke. Estrogen replacement is a crap shoot—it helps some women, and makes others worse.

Evaluate your medication options. Ongoing use of NSAIDs prevents attacks in 20 percent of migraine sufferers. Stronger doses that require a prescription are even more effective. Beta-blockers, otherwise used for treating high blood pressure, angina, and heart rhythm irregularities, also reduce the frequency of this disorder. I prescribe them for virtually all my patients with migraines. But these drugs slow the heart rate, lower blood pressure, can cause fatigue, and diminish your sex drive. Avoid them, too, if you have chronic lung disease.

The FDA has also approved calcium channel blockers such as Isoptin (verapamil) for this purpose, as well as the antiseizure drug Depakote (divalproex) used by epileptics. But women should not use the latter in their childbearing years. The older tricyclic antidepressants such as Elavil (amitriptyline) can prevent migraine, too. Vitamin B_2 (riboflavin) in a 400-milligram daily dose has been reported to reduce the number of migraine attacks. There is no downside and it's worth a try.

A group of cardiac drugs, the angiotensin-converting enzyme (ACE) inhibitors, is under investigation for the possible prevention of migraine. These drugs, of which Capoten (captopril) is the prototype, are generally safe for treating high blood pressure and heart failure. However, it's still too early to recommend them for migraine prevention.

Eradicate a bug. Some migraine sufferers who harbor *Helicobacter pylori* in their stomachs (the bacterium associated with ulcers and stomach cancer) report a decreased frequency of attacks after this bacterium is eliminated by antibiotics. It's a good idea to get rid of *H. pylori* anyway, even if you don't have migraine (see page 34 and 186).

HERE'S WHAT'S NEW

Botox injection is new approach that's received considerable hype. The same botulinum toxin that can kill you if you ingest it in tainted foods is diluted many millions of times and injected directly into the scalp muscles and paralyzes them. This leaves them unable to respond to the nerve signals that throw them into spasm. (The same toxin also eliminates unsightly wrinkles when injected into the face and ends excessive perspiration in the armpits—see pages 38 and 375.) It's worth a try if other therapy is not effective. Remember, however, that these injections are both costly and short-lived. They must be repeated every few months.

An alternative treatment receiving attention for both prevention and treatment of migraine is feverfew. This herb has been approved in Canada for migraine prevention. Several reports attest to its effectiveness. There's no harm trying it unless you're pregnant. Make sure the preparation you're using has the word "parthenolide" written on the label.

THE BOTTOM LINE

Frova is the most recent FDA-approved medication for migraines. Ask your doctor about it. Botox and feverfew may be worth trying if nothing else works for your migraines. However, the best solution is to try to prevent it. Dietary and lifestyle changes can help. If you do have an attack, several powerful over-the-counter drugs can provide relief; if they don't, ask your doctor to prescribe triptan.

MITRAL VALVE PROLAPSE

· · · · · · · · ·

Antibiotics May Be Passé

ANY TYPE OF CARDIAC DIAGNOSIS can generate fear and anxiety. Mitral valve prolapse (MVP), the most common heart valve "abnormality," affecting between 5 and 20 percent of the population, should be an exception. It's usually not worth worrying about.

The mitral valve lies between the heart's left atrium (which receives fresh, oxygenated blood from the lungs) and the left ventricle (which pumps that blood out to the rest of the body). When the left ventricle is empty after its last contraction, and ready to receive blood from the left atrium, the mitral valve opens, allowing the blood to flow into it. When the left atrium has emptied, the mitral valve closes, sealing itself off.

The mitral valve has two flaps, or leaflets. In MVP, one or both of them are too large so that the valve doesn't close properly with each heartbeat. This imperfect closing, or prolapse, causes the valve to balloon back slightly into the left atrium when the heart contracts and creates a "click" that the doctor can hear through a stethoscope. In some cases of MVP, some blood may leak back into the left atrium.

Typically diagnosed in women (between ages 20 and 40) when the doctor hears the "click," MVP is confirmed by an echocardiogram. MVP often produces no symptoms and is generally harmless, although some patients do experience fleeting "panic attacks" that make their heart pound and send them into a cold sweat. Others may experience mild shortness of breath on exertion, or occasional pain or palpitations.

HERE'S WHAT'S NEW

Until recently, doctors used to prescribe antibiotics before dental work or any other invasive procedure to all patients with MVP. This was to prevent infection of the mitral valve in the mistaken belief that its prolapse creates a potential breeding ground for any bacteria that enters the bloodstream. We now know that this is not the case. *You do not need antibiotics for MVP unless you also have a significant leak (or regurgitation) across the valve, something the echocardiogram will clearly indicate.*

If you have been diagnosed with MVP, remember that you are not a "cardiac" and do not have a "heart condition." Take the following steps to manage your health and ease symptoms:

Stay active. Do not be afraid to participate in a regular fitness program. It will make you feel better.

Avoid stimulants. Weight-reduction pills and frequent use of nasal decongestants, as well as too much caffeine and sweets can accelerate the heart rate, induce anxiety, and give you palpitations.

Curb panic attacks. The right therapy can cut the frequency and severity of these attacks by 60 to 80 percent. Ask your doctor which antidepressants, anti-anxiety drugs, or benzodiazepines are best for you.

Make sure of the diagnosis. Your doctor should establish the exact nature of any heart rhythm disturbance causing your palpitations, irregular heartbeats, or pounding of the heart. This can be done with a long-term portable monitor if the distrubance is not present on your electrocardiogram in the doctor's office. Several medications are available to control these rhythm disturbances once they have been identified. Remember, however, that the purpose of treating them is to make you comfortable. They are rarely a threat to you, and reassurance is the best medication of all.

THE BOTTOM LINE

Unless your mitral valve prolapse is accompanied by significant leak across the valve, no treatment is necessary. Antibiotics are no longer prescribed prophylactically either.

MULTIPLE SCLEROSIS

· · · · · · · · ·

Start Treatment Right Away

MULTIPLE SCLEROSIS **(MS)** is a chronic, progressive disease of the nervous system for which there is no cure. It is the most common nervous system disorder in young adults and affects more than 2 million people worldwide, women more often than men. It's five times more common in temperate zones than in the tropics. If a close relative has MS, you're at least 10 times more likely to develop it, too.

Symptoms of the disease are caused by the random denuding of the nerves, much like the fraying of an electrical wire. Where the sheath that insulates the nerves and maintains their normal function becomes inflamed and is ultimately destroyed, various signs and symptoms ensue. The most common are the sudden onset of visual problems, slurred speech, trouble walking, numbness here and there, vertigo, clumsiness, trembling, loss of bladder control, seizures, paralysis—in short, malfunction wherever the involved nerves are located. Over the years, as more nerves are affected, patients become progressively disabled. However, 10 percent of patients remain stable over the years.

The cause of MS remains a mystery, but most doctors believe it's an autoimmune disease in which the body's defense mechanisms mistakenly attack and destroy healthy tissues, in this case, the nerve sheaths.

Treatments for MS are either directed against specific symptoms or act on the immune system to slow the progress of the disease. "Suppressive" medications include steroids, Copaxone (glatiramer acetate), Avonex (interferon beta), and others that also are used to treat other autoimmune diseases, for example, rheumatoid arthritis.

After doctors diagnose MS, they usually wait for at least one more attack before starting treatment. (In fact, many hesitate to make the diagnosis until two attacks have occurred.) The rationale for this conservative approach is that because no cure exists anyway, one should delay drug treatment until the symptoms recur or are troublesome (symptoms of MS typically wax and wane).

HERE'S WHAT'S NEW

New research suggests that the sooner suppressive therapy is started, the more beneficial it is over the long-term. In keeping with these findings, the FDA has approved the use of Avonex, the most widely prescribed MS drug, to be given at the first evidence of the disease. Avonex belongs to the interferon beta family and is administered once a week by injection.

THE BOTTOM LINE

If you've had MS for some time, chances are you're already taking one of the drugs previously listed. However, if you have experienced the first symptoms of the disease and are waiting for another move before starting therapy, you should probably start taking Avonex *now*. Early treatment may make a difference in the long run.

New Discoveries on the Horizon

MULTIPLE SCLEROSIS is a tragic disease that inspires researchers to continue their search for more effective ways to slow its progress, minimize its symptoms, and hopefully find a cure.

HERE'S WHAT'S NEW

A new class of drugs has been developed to treat MS based on the belief that it is an autoimmune disorder. Current MS drugs act on the harmful immune cells *after* they've left the blood and begun to attack vulnerable nerve tissues. The new ones, the prototype of which is Antegren (natalizumab), actually prevent these cells from leaving the bloodstream and attacking their target. (This unique action is expected to be of use in treating other autoimmune disorders such as inflammatory bowel disease.) Initial experience with Antegren in MS have revealed as much as a 93 percent reduction in new nerve lesions and 50 percent fewer relapses.

Researchers, in yet another approach to treating this disease are evaluating the cholesterol-lowering statin drugs—Zocor (simvastatin), Pravachol (pravastatin), Lipitor (atorvastatin), and Lescol (fluvastatin).

In a small trial involving 28 MS patients ages 18 to 55, a daily dose of Zocor for 6 months decreased the number of their relapses from 43 to 32 percent. There were also fewer new nerve lesions detected in brain scans. This drug apparently inhibits several different immune responses and markers of inflammation characteristic of MS. Other statins showed similar effects, but they were less marked.

It's still too early to recommend taking statin drugs for MS. More studies are needed—and indeed have begun—to ensure they aren't harmful over the long term. However, the initial observations are encouraging. If you have MS, be on the lookout for the follow-up reports on this research.

As their disease progresses, MS patients often have trouble understanding new information and remembering it. It's not as bad as having Alzheimer's disease, but still distressing. So researchers wondered whether MS patients might also benefit from medication that helps Alzheimer's. They found that Aricept (donepezil), medication that enhances memory modestly by increasing the concentration of neurotransmitters that help transfer messages among different parts of the brain, did help more than 65 percent of MS patients tested. Other objective test scores were also measurably improved. However, the drug had no effect on how quickly the disease's process.

A research team at the Oregon Health and Science University studied 69 patients with MS and reported that exercise and yoga improved their fatigue—a major complaint of MS patients.

THE BOTTOM LINE

The rate at which MS patients get progressively worse is unpredictable. For example, I have several whose symptoms remain barely discernible for years; in others, their debilitation continues without letup. However, if you have MS, take comfort in the fact that research is proceeding at a furious pace. New theories, new drugs, and new approaches are being reported virtually every day. I have described some that may make a difference. Don't hesitate to try those your neurologist recommends, bearing in mind that new ones are always on the way. One of them will surely help you. In the meantime, stay physically and mentally active—and keep your spirits up.

OSTEOPOROSIS

· · · · · · · · ·

Prevent It with Vitamin D

THE TERM "OSTEOPOROSIS" MEANS POROUS BONES that have become thin and fragile due to loss of their calcium. The resulting fractures, especially of the hips, spine, and wrist, are a major health problem in the United States.

Twenty-eight million Americans, 80 percent of whom are women, either have significant osteoporosis or are on the way to developing it. One of every two females and one of eight men over 50 will fracture at least one bone in her or his lifetime. This translates into 300,000 hip fractures (80,000 of them in men), 700,000 vertebral fractures (accounting for the loss of height and the so-called dowager's hump in some older women), 250,000 wrist fractures, and more than 300,000 broken bones elsewhere in the body every year.

Pain, suffering, and death aside, these fractures add up to a staggering $14 billion in hospital and nursing home bills annually.

You can control most, but not all, of the risk factors of osteoporosis. Here are some important ones that you can't do much about:

Sex. Women are at much greater risk than men because their bones are thinner to begin with, and they lose calcium more easily because of the hormonal changes at menopause.

Age. The older you are, the more likely you are to have osteoporosis.

Body size. Short women with thinner bones are at greater risk than bigger and heavier ones.

Ethnicity. Caucasian and Asian women are more prone than African-American and Latina women.

Family history. If your parents had osteoporosis, chances are that you will develop it, too.

You can reduce this greater vulnerability by taking the following steps:

Exercise. Regular weight-bearing exercise in which you work against gravity—such as walking, stair climbing, dancing, and hiking—is great for your bones and helps them retain their calcium.

Eat more calcium. One of the most effective ways to keep your bones strong as you age is to consume lots of calcium, a mineral present in a wide variety in foods. The best known dietary sources are leafy vegetables and nonfat dairy products, but there are many others. And if you can't or won't eat these foods, you can get the calcium you need in supplements.

Take vitamin D. Your stomach must have enough vitamin D to absorb dietary calcium. In the elderly, who may not get enough vitamin D, doctors recommend supplements of 400 to 800 international units (IU) a day.

If you are menopausal and want to know if you have osteoporosis, you should have an x-ray examination called bone densitometry regularly every couple of years after your periods have ended.

If densitometry reveals evidence of osteoporosis, there are several medications that can halt its progress—and sometimes even reverse it. Not so long ago, women had only estrogen replacement therapy to strengthen their bones. The downside to hormone replacement therapy (especially the risk of cancer) outweighs the benefits (see page 244). Happily, there are effective alternatives. The main ones include:

Actonel (risedronate). A 35-milligram tablet taken once a week increases the calcium content of your bones, and slows or arrests bone loss and reduces the risk of fractures.

Fosamax (alendronate). A 70-milligram tablet a week is all you need to reverse bone loss. This drug also is approved for preventing osteoporosis, at 35 milligrams per week.

Evista (raloxifene) belongs to a class of drugs called selective estrogen receptor modulators. Like estrogen, Evista improves osteoporosis and reduces the incidence of fractures. However, because it blocks the action of estrogen on breast cells, it does not lead to breast cancer and it may actually reduce that risk. Evista's main downside is that it occasionally causes blood clots in the veins (see page 181).

Calcitonin. This non-sex hormone is prescribed for women who are at least 5 years into menopause, usually in the form of a nasal spray. It slows bone loss and reduces the risk of spinal fractures.

Any of these medications are standard therapy for osteoporosis, and they're all moderately effective. However, as with any drug, they may have adverse effects, and some of them are expensive.

HERE'S WHAT'S NEW

Doctors at the University of Cambridge in England have found that high doses of oral vitamin D (the British study focused on vitamin D_3, known as cholecalciferol) taken every 4 months reduce the risk of osteoporosis in men and women between ages 65 and 85—at a cost of less than $2 a year! We're talking 100,000 IU per pill, not the 800 IU in the usual daily dose. Patients so treated had an overall fracture incidence of less than 22 percent and had 33 percent fewer breaks in the most vulnerable bones, such as the hip, wrist, and spine.

THE BOTTOM LINE

I have no experience with such high doses of vitamin D, but other doctors have—usually for the treatment of multiple sclerosis, other autoimmune diseases, and some cases of advanced prostate cancer. But given the dramatic effect of just three doses a year, this therapy should be seriously considered for all men and postmenopausal women with osteoporosis or those vulnerable to it.

The main adverse effects of excessive vitamin D are nausea, gastric irritation, and too much calcium in the blood. High blood calcium levels can harm the kidneys and the heart. Although in this particular study, which involved more than 2,000 people, the 100,000 IU dose apparently was well-tolerated. If you decide to try this treatment, make sure to check your blood calcium level every couple of months. If it rises above 11 milligrams/deciliter, forgo the next dose of vitamin D.

A Fortunate Drug Discovery

OSTEOPOROSIS is sometimes so severe that the brittle and porous bones resemble Swiss cheese and are at constant risk for bone fracture at the slightest provocation. In such cases, a new drug may make all the difference.

HERE'S WHAT'S NEW

The latest medication is an injectable form of human parathyroid hormone, a naturally occurring compound that controls the absorption and loss of calcium from bone. The drug's chemical name is teriparatide; its brand name is Forteo. It dramatically reverses the damage of osteoporosis, increasing the thickness of bone and reconnecting the pieces by activating cells that actually make bone. In one study of postmenopausal women with severe osteoporosis, Forteo reduced spine fractures by 65 percent and other fractures by 53 percent.

Forteo is not nearly as convenient as the other anti-osteoporosis medications. You must inject yourself every day for a year and a half (the FDA has placed a 24-month limit on the drug's use) with pen-like needles, much like those used by diabetics. Some rats injected with high doses of Forteo developed a rare bone cancer, but this finding was not observed in any of the 2,000 men and women who used the drug for up to a year and a half.

THE BOTTOM LINE

Forteo should be used only as last resort and only for the most severe cases. For severe cases of osteoporosis, in which the risk of fracture is great, Forteo can save the day. If you have been disabled by osteoporosis and are suffering recurrent fractures, discuss the drug with your doctor. Forteo is not for anyone who has had previous radiation therapy of the bones, Paget's disease of bone, or a cancer that has spread to the bone. Nor should it be given to growing children or young adults.

OVARIAN CANCER

· · · · · · · · ·

Know Your Risk Factors

OVARIAN CANCER strikes one in every 55 women. More than 25,000 will develop it sometime during the next year and almost 15,000 will die. Although 95 percent of ovarian cancers can be cured if detected before they have spread beyond the ovary, the actual 5-year survival rate is less than 50 percent. That's because most of these malignancies are diagnosed too late. The main reason is that the ovaries are situated deep inside the pelvis and are not easy to feel and there is no single reliable screening test for early detection.

So you've got to look for ovarian cancer—very carefully using several different methods—in order to find it. Unfortunately, doctors don't recommend this kind of in-depth exam unless their patients are specifically vulnerable to the disease.

The red flags of ovarian cancer are persistent and unexplained painful intercourse, bloating, extreme fatigue, unusual vaginal bleeding, a feeling of pressure in the pelvis, swelling of the abdomen, and chronic stomach pain, gas, or indigestion. But frankly, when these are present, the tumor has probably already spread. So it's better to look for it when you're still feeling well.

The following women are at special risk for ovarian cancer:

- Postmenopausal women in their late fifties and sixties. If they've been taking estrogen replacement therapy, their chances are more than doubled.

- Females of North American or North European descent, particularly Ashkenazi Jews (from central and eastern Europe).

- Women who test positive for mutations of the BRCA1 or BRCA2 genes. The presence of the BRCA1 mutation confers a 20 to 40 percent chance of developing ovarian cancer during your lifetime (and/or a 50 to 85 percent likelihood of breast cancer); the BRCA2 mutation carries a 15 to 20 percent chance of cancer of the ovaries (and a 55 to 85 percent likelihood of breast cancer). You should be tested for both of these genes if you have a family history (mother, sister, or daughter) of either ovarian or breast malignancy. (About 5 percent of Ashkenazi women have mutations of these genes.)

- Women who have had a previous malignancy of the uterus, colon, or breast.

- Women with a family history (mother, sister, or daughter) of ovarian, breast, uterine, or colon cancer have an increased lifetime chance of developing ovarian cancer. If one such relative had ovarian cancer, your risk is 1 in 20; with two or more, it's 1 in 14.

- Women who have never had a baby or who had their first one after age 30, whose periods started before age 12, and/or whose menopause didn't set in until well after age 50 have more ovarian cancer. The greater the number of periods you've had during your life, the greater the risk.

- Women who have used fertility drugs such as Clomid (clomiphene) unsuccessfully.

HERE'S WHAT'S NEW

You are at *reduced* risk for ovarian cancer if your tubes were tied, or you used oral contraceptives for at least 5 years, or if you breastfed your infant (because periods usually stop during breastfeeding).

If for any reason you and/or your doctor think there's even the *slightest* possibility of ovarian cancer (family history, physical findings, puzzling symptoms—remember, you don't have to be sure, just suspicious) your doctor should perform the following procedures:

- A bimanual pelvic exam via the vagina *and the rectum* to feel the ovaries.

- A blood test called the CA 125 to measure the level of a protein that is elevated in the presence of ovarian cancer. (This same protein may also be increased by uterine [endometrial] and other cancers; and it also may be falsely elevated in healthy women.) However, CA 125 reading alone is not diagnostic, one way or another.

- More and more MRIs and CT scans of the pelvis are being performed for ovarian cancer screening. Unfortunately, they are expensive. You may also have a transvaginal sonogram (the sonic probe is inserted into the vagina) or a color ultrasound Doppler (which looks at the blood vessels in the ovary), both of which can detect ovarian cysts and are especially useful when combined with the CA 125 analysis. However, they can miss early ovarian tumors.

If you have a positive family history, one or more of these tests should be done every 6 months, starting at age 35. It sounds like overkill, but it's worth it. In the final analysis, when the diagnosis of ovarian cancer seems like a real possibility, laparoscopy or surgery may be the only way to establish the diagnosis with certainty. Any suspicious tissue should be biopsied.

There are several ways to treat ovarian cancer, and new ones are in the works. Know all your options before you commit yourself to any particular one. If you have any questions or doubts, get a second opinion. You may also call the National Cancer Institute at (800) 4-CANCER or log on to the Internet and ask an expert at a Web site such as www.cancersource.com, www.cancerfacts.com, or www.oncology.com. The outlook for ovarian cancer depends on its stage when discovered. Regardless, the tumor should always be removed, followed by chemotherapy with or without radiation.

Women at high risk for ovarian cancer often ask me whether they should have their ovaries removed while they're still healthy. Here's what I tell them: If you have two or more first-degree relatives, or first- and second-degree relatives with ovarian cancer, you should be examined for the BRCA1 and BRCA2 gene mutations. If you test positive, I recommend prophylactic removal of the ovaries (oophrectomy) unless you plan to have more children. This surgery can be done by video laparoscopy (without a major incision), leaving the uterus intact. You should then take hormone replacement therapy at the lowest possible dose for the shortest possible time. Interestingly, 2 percent of women who undergo such prophylactic oophrectomy later develop a malignancy in the lining of the abdomen (the peritoneum) that resembles ovarian cancer. So even after your ovaries have been removed, have a physical exam and CA 125 test once or twice a year. A CA 125 reading, while not reliable as a screen in presumably healthy women, is very useful in evaluating the success of therapy for ovarian cancer.

Chalk up another plus for aspirin: According to recent research, aspirin may decrease the risk of ovarian cancer by as much as 40 percent. If you're worried about a family history of the disease, it's well worth asking your doctor whether you should be taking prophylactic aspirin.

THE BOTTOM LINE

Know your risk factors for ovarian cancer and do what you can to minimize them. Daily aspirin can cut your risk. Also, having a hysterectomy, taking birth control pills over the long term, or breastfeeding your babies may also reduce your chances of developing this cancer.

Always suspect ovarian cancer if you develop a constellation of unexplained symptoms in the pelvis or abdomen—gas, bloating, fatigue, a change in your menstrual pattern, stomach pain or distension, or pain or pressure in the pelvis. But remember that this cancer is often silent and you have to look for it.

The most useful, although by no means foolproof, steps to take are regular, careful rectovaginal exams by your gynecologist, and a vaginal ultrasound or pelvic CT or MRI. If you're at high risk for ovarian cancer, consider prophylactic removal of both ovaries after you've had your family. And, once again, remember the aspirin.

OVERWEIGHT

· · · · · · · · ·

The Latest News about the Atkins Diet

MANY THOUSANDS OF AMERICANS eager to lose weight are following the high-fat, low-carbohydrate Atkins Diet, a regimen that has been for many years anathema to the American Heart Association (AHA) and to most cardiologists. Countless studies over the years have shown that eating large amounts of saturated fat and cholesterol for long periods of time is associated with a higher incidence of heart attacks and strokes. However, Dr. Atkins continued to insist steadfastly, until his untimely death in April 2003, that his diet neither raises cholesterol nor causes arteriosclerosis. In addition, he asserted that eating all the butter, cream, fatty meat, and bacon that your heart desires (no pun intended) actually improves the fat profile of the blood. He explained it all by the impact of his diet on insulin sensitivity and the breakdown of stored fat in the body tissues. In Atkins's view, carbohydrate is the villain, not fat.

HERE'S WHAT'S NEW

This past year the Atkins Diet was evaluated in several studies conducted by "establishment" scientists and reported in mainstream publications such as the *New England Journal of Medicine*. The results from one study, done at Duke University (supported by an unrestricted grant from the Atkins Foundation), are similar to all the others. The researchers randomly assigned 120 overweight volunteers either to the Atkins Diet (carbohydrate intake less than 20 grams a day, with 60 percent of calories coming from fat, supplemented by flaxseed, borage, and fish oils) or to the AHA's Step 1 Diet (total fat intake less than 30 percent of daily calories).

The researchers found that after 6 months the Atkins dieters lost 31 pounds; those on the AHA Diet dropped 20 pounds. But those on the Atkins Diet preferred it to the AHA Diet. Most impressive, however, was the finding that HDL levels (the "good" cholesterol) *increased* by 11 percent on the supposedly dangerous Atkins diet, but remained unchanged on the AHA Diet; triglyceride levels (another risk factor for heart disease) *decreased* by 49 percent in the Atkins group, but fell by only 22 percent in the AHA group. LDL levels (the "bad" cholesterol) did not change in either group, but in those eating à la Atkins, the cholesterol was altered to a form less likely to clog the arteries. Finally, the Atkins Diet resulted in a 49 percent drop in VLDL levels (the cholesterol type most strongly linked to heart disease) and only 17 percent with the AHA Diet.

About a month after Dr. Atkins died, two more studies (one of 6 months duration, the other a year) confirmed the results of the earlier research—that is, the high-fat, low-carbohydrate Atkins Diet helps people lose weight without adversely affecting their cholesterol profile. However, at the end of 1 year, Atkins dieters regained about one-third of the pounds lost, whereas the AHA group regained only one-fifth of their weight.

THE BOTTOM LINE

At first glance, it would appear that the Atkins Diet is preferable to that currently recommended by cardiologists. However, the AHA points out that virtually all these studies were of short duration. Cardiologists remain concerned about the *long-term* consequences of eating large amounts of saturated fat. The AHA continues to warn us not to abandon a low-fat regimen and to follow a diet rich in fruits, vegetables, whole grains, lean meat, fish, poultry, and low-fat dairy products. In addition, the concern is not only about vascular disease, but the possibility that saturated fat raises the risk of breast cancer in women.

For all these reasons, until more long-term findings become available, here's what I'm telling my patients: The Atkins Diet is a safe, even healthy, short-term way to lose weight. I have no objection to them trying it for up to 6 months to lose weight. However, if their cholesterol level is high or they are otherwise at risk for vascular disease, I recommend that they also take a statin or other cholesterol-lowering drug—just to be on the safe side.

WHAT THE DOCTOR ORDERED?

GASTRIC BYPASS SURGERY FOR OVERWEIGHT
DIABETICS ● Weight is a national obsession. I'd be a rich man today if I'd had the foresight to buy stock in a weight-scale manufacturing company. Do you know anyone who doesn't weigh them-

selves every day? My wife, my kids, and I all do. We even have two scales, one of which is set a little lower for when the fit of our clothes suggests that we've gained a pound or two but we don't want to admit it. Do you know anyone who isn't dieting, or who is satisfied with his or her weight, or who doesn't "need" to lose "just a few pounds?"

Ironically, this preoccupation with weight is usually not because people worry that being fat is dangerous to their health. It's mostly for the sake of appearance. In our culture, thin is considered beautiful; fat is not.

The truth is we are in the midst of a dangerous epidemic of obesity. Two-thirds of us weigh more than we should, and we are becoming fatter by the minute. Significant overweight leaves you vulnerable to heart disease, stroke, several cancers, osteo-arthritis, sleep apnea, high blood pressure, urinary incontinence, and diabetes.

With rare exceptions, overweight is the result of consuming more calories than we burn. Mind you, some medical disorders, such as a low-functioning thyroid gland and other hormonal disturbances, can cause or contribute to it, but they're just drops in the bucket.

How do you know if you're really overweight? Most people look in the mirror or decide on the basis of how their clothes fit. Doctors used to refer to life insurance height-weight tables, but few still do. Most men and women, patients and doctors alike, use other parameters such as the Body Mass Index (BMI) and other mathematical calculations to determine optimal weight. (Calculate your BMI with the following formula: BMI = your weight [in kilograms] divided by your height expressed in square meters.) Morbid obesity is defined as more than 100 pounds in excess of ideal body weight or a BMI of 40 or higher. How weight is distributed is also important: Fat thighs are safer than big bellies.

Everyone—your own doctor, your favorite movie star, and followers of the late Dr. Atkins—has a "foolproof" way to lose weight. Pharmaceutical manufacturers regularly churn out a succession of drugs "guaranteed" to take the pounds off—until they're forced to pull them from the market because too many people have suffered complications, even died, as a result of using them. Herbal gurus have their own armamentarium, including ephedra, which we now know is dangerous (see page 283).

Although few if any weight-reduction treatments are effective for any length of time, one "last resort" approach—gastric bypass surgery—does work. Just ask (and look at) Al Roker, the genial NBC weatherman. He's a shadow of his former self, and loving every minute of it. Like him, more and more obese people are choosing this option.

In the most common gastric bypass operation, called Roux-en-Y, the stomach is stapled and divided. It's done laparoscopically, meaning the surgeon inserts instruments through tiny abdominal incisions. The procedure seals off most of the stomach leaving a small pouch at the top that receives the food you eat. Since the pouch can't hold very much, you eat less and lose weight—an average loss of 50 to 60 percent of excess pounds. Your appetite shrinks too, as does your taste for many foods. People who undergo this procedure require supplements because their stomachs no longer can absorb enough iron, calcium, and vitamin B_{12}.

Although gastric bypass operations are normally well-tolerated, they are as risky as any surgery because of infection, clots, pain, and (rarely) cardiac complications. Most patients remain in the hospital for 3 to 4 days after the procedure.

One after effect of the surgery is "dumping syndrome," characterized by such symptoms as nausea, vomiting, diarrhea, abdominal cramps, flushing, and palpitations. It occurs after eating sugar because the "stomach" area in which sugar is digested is now much smaller. So sugar enters the small intestine without having been properly digested. The undigested sugar causes symptoms that resemble those of lactose intolerance, in which undigested lactose remains in the gut because of a deficiency of the enzyme lactase. Like lactose deficiency, dumping syndrome is unpleasant but not dangerous.

HERE'S WHAT'S NEW • The weight loss after gastric bypass surgery often reverses type 2 (adult-onset) diabetes. If the weight loss is maintained, the disease can, in effect, be *cured*.

Doctors at the University of Pittsburgh studied 192 men and women with type 2 diabetes who had a mean weight loss of 97 pounds after laparoscopic Roux-en-Y gastric bypass surgery. Diabetes disappeared in 73 percent of them and improved in 24 percent. Only 3 percent had no change in their diabetic status. The least impressive results were seen in patients with high insulin requirements or who'd had the disease for a very long time. But even when the diabetes was not cured, the patient required much less insulin to control blood glucose levels.

THE BOTTOM LINE • If you're overweight, and especially if you have a family history of diabetes, it's important for you to lose weight to prevent developing the disease. The best way to do that is to eat less and exercise more. But if you have type 2 diabetes, are morbidly obese (weigh 100 or more pounds than you should, or have a BMI of 40 or higher), consider gastric bypass surgery. A successful operation may improve your health substantially and even eliminate your diabetes. ◦

Ephedra—Avoid It

HERBS ARE CLASSIFIED as "food supplements" and not regulated by the FDA. That means you can buy and consume them in unlimited quantities.

Many doctors, including myself, think that's a mistake. Why? Herbs are potent, which, after all, is why they're used. Some are potentially as toxic as the more than 100 drugs for which you need a doctor's prescription that are derived from herbs. Most of them are safe in small doses, but an overdose is dangerous. The best example is digitalis, extracted from the foxglove plant. It's an important and powerful drug that strengthens the heart and controls an abnormal cardiac rhythm. However, if you take too much, the heart rhythm first "goes crazy" and then the heart stops. Doctors have a great deal of respect for this powerful herb; they prescribe it only in very small doses and then monitor patients closely. For these reasons the herb isn't sold in health food stores—and neither should many others.

The herb ephedra (its Chinese name is *ma huang*) is a case in point. Until recently it was freely available without a doctor's prescription in health food stores and was widely used for weight loss and as a stimulant. It contains ephedrine, which doctors formerly prescribed as a decongestant, stimulant, and antiasthmatic but have largely abandoned because of its adverse effects. Ironically, after doctors stopped prescribing it several years ago, it found its way onto the shelves of health food stores, where it became a big seller in the weight-reduction business. Its continued use has been the subject of heated arguments between the medical profession and the manufacturers.

The first break in this war was the recommendation that warnings be placed on labels limiting the dose of the drug. That left the burden on the user. Not a good idea, according to many doctors.

HERE'S WHAT'S NEW

According to recent research, taking more than 32 milligrams of ephedra triples the chance of having a brain hemorrhage (stroke) within 3 days.

In addition, researchers at the San Francisco Medical Center studied the available data on the use of ephedra ever published in the *Annals of Internal Medicine*, the official journal of the American College of Physicians. They found that in the year 2001, although ephedra accounted for less than 1 percent of all herbal supplement sales in the United States, it was responsible for 62 percent of all reported herb-related complications. (Who knows how many adverse effects were not reported?)

Ephedra's most dangerous adverse effects are high blood pressure and increased heart rate, which can and do result in heart attacks and strokes. Less serious consequences are anxiety and insomnia. The researchers conclude from these data that the risk posed by taking ephedra is 200 times greater than that from all other tested herbal supplements combined! Ephedra is 100 times more dangerous than kava (which has been banned in several countries) and 720 times more dangerous than ginkgo biloba. With all the other threats to your health that are beyond your control, you need ephedra like you need a hole in the head. Researchers conclude that ephedra should either be banned or only be taken under close supervision. Practically speaking, that means making it a prescription drug available only if your doctor thinks you need it.

The ephedra saga has been evolving rapidly. State after state has banned its sale. Finally, the FDA removed it from the market entirely.

THE BOTTOM LINE

No matter why you take ephedra, whether to lose weight or to increase your energy levels, there are better and safer ways to accomplish your goal, especially if you have heart trouble or high blood pressure.

PARKINSON'S DISEASE

· · · · · · · · ·

Bold Approaches to a Shaky Prognosis

WHEN YOU'RE BASICALLY HEALTHY, except for a minor illness now and then, you're apt to have very little interest in news about treating a condition with which you don't identify. But patients with terminal cancer, or crippling disease such as Lou Gehrig's disease, or multiple sclerosis, or the 1.5 million victims of Parkinson's disease, are desperate for a breakthrough that can save them.

Parkinson's affects 1 in every 100 men and women over age 65 making it the fourth most common "neurodegenerative" disease of the elderly. It starts at the average age of 57 and, along with Alzheimer's disease, is one of the most dreaded afflictions.

James Parkinson, an English physician, first described this disease in 1817, referring to it as "shaking palsy." The first treatment breakthrough did not come until about 50 years ago when scientists examining the brains of patients who had died with Parkinson's disease found an area of the brain called the *substantia nigra* deficient in cells that produce a chemical called dopamine. This is a neurotransmitter that sends messages from one part of the brain to another. They concluded that the symptoms of Parkinson's disease are due to dopamine deficiency. The man who made this key observation won the Nobel Prize in medicine.

Unfortunately, replacing the missing dopamine doesn't cure the disease because the brain is very selective about what it allows to enter it. That's how it protects itself from potentially harmful chemicals circulating in the bloodstream. Researchers found that a naturally occurring substance called dopa, related to but different from dopamine, could penetrate this "blood-brain" barrier. However, the amounts necessary to be of any help were otherwise so toxic that it could not be used.

Enter Dr. George Cotzias, a neurologist friend of mine working at Cornell Medical School some 40 years ago. He found that modifying dopa into levodopa did cross the barrier into the brain where it was converted to dopamine and improved the symptoms of the disease. To this day, levodopa remains the basic treatment for millions of patients with Parkinson's disease. Unfortunately, levodopa improves symptoms only partially. What's more, the longer you take it and the higher the dose, the greater its debilitating side effects—uncontrollable jerky movements, elevated blood pressure, hallucinations, delirium, and decreased effectiveness.

HERE'S WHAT'S NEW

Researchers at the Institute of Neurosciences at Frenchay Hospital in Bristol, England, treated five patients suffering from advanced Parkinson's disease with growth factor delivered in GDNF (glial cell-line derived neurotrophic factor) injected daily *directly into the brain through a special pump*! This technique has shown promise in rats and primates. These injections were found to be safe in humans, and they improved symptoms and slowed the progression of the disease in all five patients. Larger trials are now being conducted.

Gene therapy is another important potential breakthrough currently being explored. Monkeys whose brains were rendered deficient in dopamine and who had developed symptoms of Parkinson's disease were injected with a virus that was engineered to carry a gene that stimulates the formation of dopamine-producing cells. Three months later these monkeys were found to be making normal amounts of neurotransmitter and had lost their Parkinson's symptoms. More recently, at the Weill Cornell Medical Center in New York, my colleagues in neurosurgery have injected genes into the brain of a severely disabled Parkinson's patient. He tolerated the procedure well and is being observed for clinical improvements. It's still too early to tell whether he has been helped, but the researchers plan to perform more such injections in the months to come.

In the meantime, other medications new and old can help ease the burden of Parkinson's. Here's the current status of therapies for this disease:

Levodopa. Levodopa is still the basic drug for Parkinson's. However, because of its adverse effects, many doctors delay prescribing it for as long as possible. Several less toxic drugs can be used instead in the early stages. Levodopa is then added when symptoms make it necessary. Combination therapy makes it possible to administer levodopa at a lower dose resulting in fewer side effects.

Agonists. The term "agonist" means that a particular chemical or drug enhances the effect of another. Dopamine agonists increase the effectiveness of whatever small amounts of dopamine the Parkinson's brain continues to produce so that patients need less levodopa.

The older dopamine agonists, Parlodel (bromocriptine) and Permax (pergolide), are less effective than the more recent ones— Maripex (pramipexole) and Requip (ropinirole). In a study of 268 patients with early Parkinson's, ropinirole was successful for 5 years without any other drugs. So if you have recently been diagnosed, consider the option of delaying levodopa and only taking a dopamine agonist.

Dopamine agonists can sometimes cause a drop in blood pressure when you stand up from a lying-down position (postural hypotension), and a variety of behavioral complications that range from confusion to delirium. Still, they're worth trying.

Symmetrel (amantadine). This dopamine agonist is widely used to treat mild cases of Parkinson's. First try it alone and, when it is no longer effective, add levodopa, whose effect it enhances. The usual dose is 100 to 300 milligrams a day. Although it's usually well tolerated, this drug can cause confusion and swelling of the legs.

Symmetrel has an interesting history. Several years ago, doctors in Russia who were evaluating its possible use in Parkinson's observed that patients given the drug who also happened to get the flu recovered more quickly from their viral infection. Further research has confirmed that Symmetrel is effective against type A influenza (see page 72). This drug, and others like it, are now part of the armamentarium against the flu—an example of how the same agent can be used in totally unrelated illnesses.

Antienzyme medications. There are enzymes in the brain that prevent neurotransmitters such as dopamine from accumulating to high, toxic levels. However, patients with Parkinson's needs all the dopamine they can produce. There are medications that prevent the usually desirable enzymatic action against dopamine and so improve Parkinson's disease. These include Eldepryl (selegiline), Tasmar (tolcapone), and Comtan (entacapone). When given for a year or two to patients who are still making some of their own dopamine early in the disease, these drugs alone may be all that's necessary. When continued along with levodopa, they can make the latter more effective in lower doses. But it's a double-edged sword because these antienzyme medications may aggravate the side effects of levodopa.

Anticholinergic agents. In addition to dopamine, the brain makes another neurotransmitter called acetylcholine. The two balance each other in healthy people because enzymes in the brain prevent either from accumulating. In Parkinson's patients whose dopamine supply is reduced but who have normal amounts of acetylcholine, the imbalance between these two neurotransmitters aggravates their symptoms. Drugs that decrease the concentration of acetylcholine can therefore be useful. Among the several such *anticholinergic agents*, the most commonly prescribed are Artane (trihexyphenidyl) and Cogentin (benztropine). They reduce tremor and muscle stiffness, but can cause dry mouth, blurred vision, constipation, urinary retention, and confusion.

Carbidopa. You can maximize the effectiveness and decrease the side effects of levodopa by adding carbidopa, a medication that prevents the breakdown of levodopa in the liver. The combination, marketed as Sinemet, is the most widely used anti-Parkinson's medication. It comes in several fixed dosages and should be taken 15 to 20 minutes before meals to make sure it is fully absorbed. Start with the lowest strength (25 milligrams of carbidopa and 100 milligrams of levodopa) and increase the dose every week or so until you're getting maximum benefit with the fewest side effects. Most patients need to raise the maintenance Sinemet dose from time to time because the brain's already limited production of dopamine continues to decline.

Sinemet can begin to lose its effectiveness after 2 to 5 years. You'll know that's happening when your symptoms worsen before your next scheduled dose. The longer you use Sinemet and the higher the dose, the more likely it is to cause side effects. So finding the right dose of Sinemet and readjusting it as necessary is critically important. When the tremor is very bad, a low dose beta-blocker such as Inderal (propranolol) can help.

THE BOTTOM LINE

Several medications can improve the symptoms of Parkinson's disease. The most important is levodopa, which is converted into the missing dopamine in the brain. Other drugs can be taken along with levodopa to enhance its action and minimize its side effects. Proper nutrition, exercise, and other lifestyle "therapies" are important to keep your muscles strong, flexible, and moving, as well as to control weight, ensure a good night's sleep, and minimize symptoms.

Certain surgical and other treatments (some are still largely experimental) can relieve specific symptoms of Parkinson's disease. For example, when involuntary movements are severe, an operation on the brain (pallidotomy) can reduce them. Deep brain stimulation of the thalamus and high-frequency stimulation of other areas also may help.

Injecting growth hormone directly into the brains of patients with Parkinson's is a new, bold, and promising step. This experiment is tangible evidence of continued attempts to conquer Parkinson's. What with stem cell and other approaches, there is reason for optimism.

PNEUMONIA

· · · · · · · · ·

Protect the Entire Family by Vaccinating the Kids

FOR YEARS, doctors have been recommending the pneumonia vaccine for anyone older than 65. They've also advised it for debilitated and vulnerable people of any age who might not survive pneumonia (for example, a man or woman with underlying lung disease, such as chronic bronchitis, in whom a pneumonia infection would be especially difficult to treat).

Adults usually are given the pneumonia vaccine every 7 years starting after age 50. However, if you receive your first dose after age 65, no further shots are required.

Pneumonia vaccine protects against 23 types of bacteria that cause pneumonia—but many more bacteria than that are lurking in the noses and throats of healthy people. These bacteria are easily spread from person to person and are dangerous to the very young, elderly, and to anyone who is chronically ill.

In 2000, a pneumonia vaccine called Prevnar was approved to protect infants and toddlers against the seven most common strains of the pneumococcus bacteria. These organisms are important and common causes of various serious infections in the very young, including pneumonia, blood infections, and meningitis. The vaccine cost $60 for each of the four doses required before age 2. This increases the previous cost of childhood immunization by about 60 percent.

HERE'S WHAT'S NEW

Here are the data in about the effectiveness of the adult pneumococcal vaccine and the newer pediatric one:

Children younger than age 2 who received the pediatric vaccine (Prevnar) were 69 percent less likely to develop strep pneumonia. In children older than age 2, the incidence dropped by 44 percent. Between ages 5 and 19, the vaccine had no significant effect.

What's most fascinating is the impact of vaccinating kids on the incidence of pneumonia in *unvaccinated adults*. Parents between ages 22 and 39 had a 32 percent decrease in pneumonia when their kids received Prevnar. The incidence of pneumonia fell by 18 percent in adults age 65 and older. Grandparents, stand up and be counted! This pediatric vaccine is protecting adults by preventing pneumonia in the kids with whom they are in close contact.

The figures for the adult pneumonia vaccine are not nearly as impressive. Although it does protect against serious meningitis and reduces the number of serious blood infections by half, it does not prevent pneumonia in the elderly, according to a recent study. A new pneumonia vaccine is needed for vulnerable adults, and it just may be that the pediatric vaccine is the answer. However, as this book goes to press, Prevnar has not been approved for us older folks.

THE BOTTOM LINE

The new pediatric pneumonia vaccine has turned out to be a blessing. Every child younger than age 2 should receive it, as recommended by health officials. It also makes it safer for us grandparents to play with our grandchildren.

As far as the adult vaccine is concerned, although it isn't as effective against pneumonia, it does protect against other serious infections. If you're older than age 65, get the one-time shot. You should also be vaccinated if you're younger and you have some other disease that makes you vulnerable to pneumonia.

PREMENSTRUAL
SYNDROME

＊＊＊＊＊＊＊＊＊

It's Chemical, Not Emotional

MOST OF THE 150 known premenstrual syndrome (PMS) symptoms that regularly strike about 80 percent of females during their childbearing years are behavioral. A few days before her period, a woman may become depressed, moody, tense, angry, or just plain ornery. She may lose interest in activities that she normally enjoys; she may not be able to concentrate, may feel exhausted, and be unable to sleep. Her muscles and joints may ache, she may feel bloated and retain fluid, her breasts become swollen and tender, and she usually has a headache, too. Almost every woman I know who has PMS also craves sweets, especially chocolate, during those few days. In about 5 percent of cases, depression and/or rage is severe enough to interfere with everyday activities. These extreme cases are termed premenstrual dysphoric disorder (PMDD).

In 1987, the American Psychiatric Association decided to designate PMS a psychiatric disorder. New research shows that PMS actually *is* in your head—but not in the way that these shrinks think!

HERE'S WHAT'S NEW

For years, PMS was considered a hormonal phenomenon. Most therapies for PMS were therefore focused on modifying hormonal levels—a little more progesterone here or some extra estrogen there. This approach has not really worked, and neither have a host of non-hormonal treatments.

Now for the big news: A recent landmark study compared hormone levels in hundreds of women with PMS of varying severity—ranging from virtually no symptoms to debilitating ones. *There was no difference in estrogen and progesterone levels, regardless of whether their symptoms were mild, severe, or non-existent.* The hormonal profile changes observed in those few days before the onset of her period, had no relation to the symptoms of PMS.

If not hormones, then what is to blame? The brain! Hormonal fluctuations present in *every* woman during that last week of the menstrual cycle probably cause a reduction in the level of serotonin—an important mood-altering substance in the brain. This key observation has shifted the emphasis on treating PMS from manipulating hormones to prescribing drugs that increase serotonin levels, specifically the selective serotonin reuptake inhibitors (SSRIs) such as Zoloft (sertraline).

Lower serotonin concentrations in the brain may account not only for the behavioral changes of PMS but for the fluid retention, bloating, and weight gain as well. During those few days before the onset of the period, the adrenal glands that sit atop the kidneys probably make too much aldosterone, a hormone that causes the body to retain salt. Aldosterone production is, in part, determined by brain serotonin levels—additional evidence of the brain's influence in PMS. In light of all these findings, treatment of PMS now focuses on brain chemistry.

Although the SSRIs are widely used for PMS, women can also take anti-anxiety medications such as BuSpar (buspirone) and Xanax (alprazolam). Vitamin and mineral supplements, notably B_6, E, and magnesium, are useful too. Regular aerobic exercise and avoiding excessive salt, alcohol, caffeine, concentrated sweets, and all tobacco may ease symptoms by favorably altering brain chemistry. Biofeedback and other stress reduction techniques, such as yoga, tai chi, and guided imagery help, too, as does the Relaxation Response (described in Dr. Herbert Benson's book of the same title). These measures all reduce stress, probably by increasing the depleted serotonin and endorphin levels. Increased light exposure reduces symptoms of depression in PMS, spend some time outdoors every day.

An herbal remedy has received a favorable review in a recent report in the *British Medical Journal*. Extracts from the fruit of the "chaste tree" *(Vitex agnus-castus)*, which grows in warm areas of Asia, Africa, and America, were found to improve symptoms of PMS. Half the women so treated were less irritable, had fewer headaches, were not as moody, and their breasts were not nearly as swollen. The active ingredients of this fruit include a mixture of iridoids and flavonoids with hormonal and neuroactive effects. Native women living in areas where the chaste tree grows have traditionally used these extracts to alleviate symptoms of PMS. This preparation is available in health food stores.

THE BOTTOM LINE

PMS has been shown to result from an abnormal response within the brain to the normal hormonal fluctuations of the menstrual cycle. The mainstays of therapy for severe cases are the SSRI antidepressants that raise low levels of serotonin in the brain. However, there are several other options, both natural and conventional. Reject the stereotype of emotional instability as the cause of PMS. It's not all *in* your head—it's just *from* it.

PROSTATE
ENLARGEMENT

• • • • • • • • •

A More Reasonable Treatment

"DOCTOR, I'D GIVE ANYTHING for a good night's sleep!" is one of the most common complaints I hear in my practice every day. All the clever radio and TV ads notwithstanding, you need more than a good mattress to ensure a long uninterrupted sleep—especially if you have a big prostate. Believe me, I know!

Men usually have no problem in their forties, but more than half have some prostate enlargement by the time they're 60, and the incidence rises in the ensuing years. By the eighth decade, 90 percent of all men have abnormally big prostates, and half of them have significant symptoms. If they're lucky, they get up only once or twice a

301

night to "go"; but for many, it's as often as every hour or two. That's something you can live with if you can get right back to sleep but if you can't, you're tired and sleepy the next day.

Insomnia isn't the only consequence of an enlarged prostate. A big gland is also prone to infection, and can lead to urinary incontinence. When they get the signal, these men have to move fast—or wear diapers.

Doctors call such enlargement "benign prostatic hyperplasia" (BPH) to indicate that the gland is not cancerous. Believe me, there's nothing benign about needing to dash to the john that often. (Incidentally, my brother John always referred to the men's room as the "Isadore.")

There's no way to prevent enlargement of the prostate gland, but you can treat its symptoms with a variety of medications. For example, drugs such as Proscar (finasteride) shrink the prostate by blocking the action of the male hormone testosterone. Herbs (red clover and saw palmetto) and a group of medications called alphablockers, such as Hytrin (terazosin) and Flomax (tamsulosin) can reduce frequency of urination.

Surgery should always be a last resort for treating a large prostate. Since enlargement of the gland is not uniform, with various areas being bigger than others, not every case is operable. Still, more than 400,000 of these operations are done every year in this country with a variety of techniques.

The most widely performed prostate surgery by far is the transurethral resection of the prostate (TURP). The excess tissue is cut away by a telescopic "hot wire loop" inserted into the urethra of the penis. Almost 90 percent of patients suitable for the procedure improve for at least 10 years, but the operation needs to be repeated in about 10 percent of cases. The surgery leaves between 1 percent and 3 percent of patients incontinent, and at least 13 percent become impotent. There are several modifications of TURP, all of which have similar long-term outcomes.

Some patients require a more extensive operation than the TURP to relieve their symptoms if the prostate is too big, or when there are stones in the urinary bladder. This "open" or "suprapubic" prostatectomy involves an incision in the lower part of the abdomen. It's a bigger operation than a TURP, but with similar long-term complications and benefits.

The prostate can also be shrunk by introducing a laser-beam or microwaves through the urethra. Their energy is converted to heat that steams away the excess prostate tissue. This technique must also occasionally be repeated.

All these methods are generally less invasive than a TURP—but also less effective. None of them is fun. That's why so many men will welcome the following news.

HERE'S WHAT'S NEW

Urologists have come up with what seems like a better way to get rid of a large prostate—sophisticated laser technique, called photoselective vaporization of the prostate (PVP). Doctors from the Weill Cornell Medical College in New York report that all patients treated with this vaporization technique had considerable and immediate reduction of their symptoms without significant complications and were discharged from the hospital within 23 hours. Doctors at the Mayo Clinic had similar results. If you need surgical correction of BPH, consider PVP first.

Side effects from this technique are fewer than those from other laser procedures because PVP does not penetrate the prostate as deeply, so the energy it generates is more focused. Since the excess prostatic mass is literally vaporized, there is less bleeding and clotting, but appears to be the easiest and most effective therapy available today.

THE BOTTOM LINE

Photoselective vaporization of the prostate is considered by many to be the most effective way currently available to reduce the size of a prostate and relieve obstruction to the outflow of urine. It has been tested for years and is sufficiently perfected to justify its use, whenever possible, for men who do not respond to medical therapy. Because of the anatomic variability of the glandular enlargement, not every case of BPH is suitable for this procedure. You should consider PVP before submitting to any other operation. A word of caution: Make sure the urologist treating you has been well trained in this technique.

PSORIASIS

· · · · · · · · · ·

The Most Significant Advance in 20 Years

MALFUNCTION OF THE IMMUNE SYSTEM can cause many different diseases—type 1 diabetes (the kind that strikes youngsters), rheumatoid arthritis, lupus, some forms of thyroid trouble and others—and new ones are constantly being identified.

It's the job of the immune system to protect you against attack by viruses, bacteria, and other enemies of human health. When it spots them, they are destroyed by a barrage of defensive reactions that destroy them. However, from time to time, certain parts of the immune system malfunction. Instead of destroying hostile and dangerous invaders, they turn against normal tissues.

Psoriasis is a case in point. This is a chronic disease that results in red, scaly, itchy patches covering different parts of the body; in some forms, the joints also become arthritic. Psoriasis is caused by the malfunction of effector T cells of the immune system, white blood cells that normally fight foreign invaders. In patients with psoriasis, these T cells mistakenly trigger other immune responses that cause the skin lesions and arthritis.

About 5.5 million people in the United States have psoriasis; in 1.5 million the skin lesions are moderate to severe. Moderate cases are those in which the lesions involve at least 2 percent of the body surface (1 percent equals the size of the palm of your hand). Severe cases affect than 10 percent of the skin surface.

Psoriasis is difficult to treat and there is no cure, but several different therapies can improve symptoms. Unfortunately, some of them are potentially toxic or stop working after a while. The agents most widely used today are Methotrex (methotrexate), Gengraf (cyclosporine), Remicade (infliximab), and Enbrel (etanercept), various ointments and PUVA (the combination of a light-sensitizing drug and ultraviolet light A). Some of these treatments are also prescribed for rheumatoid arthritis, another autoimmune disorder.

HERE'S WHAT'S NEW

The FDA has approved the drug Amevive (alefacept) to treat moderate to severe psoriasis. Amevive blocks and/or eliminates the T cells that cause psoriasis, without impairing the effectiveness of the rest of the immune system. It has been hailed as the most significant advance in the treatment of this disease in 20 years. Amevive is most useful in patients who no longer respond to conventional therapy.

Amevive is given by injection, into either a muscle or vein, once a week for 12 weeks, after which patients are reevaluated to see whether a second round of treatment is needed. The makers of Amevive estimate that about 80 percent of people who've had psoriasis for more than 15 years may benefit from this treatment.

In the studies leading to the approval of Amevive, the disease did not rebound in any cases after treatment was stopped. There were few toxic reactions, the most frequent being sore throat, dizziness, headaches, nausea, itching, and muscle ache—nonspecific symptoms common to many other medications. However, there were occasional serious complications, including blood disorders, malignancies, serious infections requiring hospitalization, and allergic reactions.

Doctors still aren't sure whether Amevive will interact with other drugs or how long patients with psoriasis should wait before using other immunosuppressant therapies after they have completed their course of treatment with this new drug.

Older people taking Amevive should be very carefully watched because it may not be as safe for them as it is for younger people. The safety and efficacy of Amevive have not been evaluated in children, so it should not be given to them. Anyone with an infection or a low T cell count (for example, those with HIV/AIDS) should not take Amevive, nor should people with any malignancy or serious infection. It's not a good idea for pregnant women and nursing mothers to use it either.

THE BOTTOM LINE

Psoriasis can be a pretty miserable condition, not only because of its symptoms but also its cosmetic impact. There are many drugs available to treat it. If your disease is severe and covers large and visible portions of your body and/or is accompanied by painful arthritis, try immunosuppressing agents such as methotrexate. If all forms of therapy fail and you do not fall into any of the categories listed above, consider Amevive. But make sure you're under the care of a rheumatologist or dermatologist experienced in treating this disease.

RICKETS

· · · · · · · · ·

Breast Milk Alone Is Not Enough
to Build Baby's Bones

BREASTFEEDING is the most natural way to feed your infant. There are many advantages to doing so—but some inconveniences, too. If you're pregnant, especially for the first time, and haven't yet made up your mind about breastfeeding, here are some of the pros and cons to help you decide, and one important new piece of information.

The greatest single advantage of breastfeeding is that your milk contains antibodies against disease that your baby has not yet had a chance to develop. Breastfeeding also saves you trouble. There are no bottles or nipples to sterilize; the milk is free (the cost of formula can add up over the months); it's always the right temperature; and it's right there when you need it. If you want to lose some of the weight you gained during your pregnancy, you're more likely to do so if you breastfeed because you expend about 100 to 150 calories a day just producing the milk.

The downside? Feeding a hungry baby takes precedence over everything else, no matter how you feel, where you are, or how tired you may be. And forget about privacy, especially if you happen to be on the subway or in some other public place. You also have to be careful about what you eat, especially if you have a family history of allergy. You must limit how much alcohol you drink, too, because it gets into your milk.

Bottlefeeding has other advantages. Your husband or babysitter can take over when you're unavailable; you don't have to bare your breasts in public; and babies who are bottlefed don't get hungry as soon after "dining" as those who are breastfed because formula takes longer to digest than breast milk.

These are the main pros and cons that I can think of, not ever having had to make that decision personally. In my opinion, they add up in favor of breastfeeding simply because protecting your child against a host of illnesses outweighs all the conveniences of bottle-feeding.

HERE'S WHAT'S NEW

Rickets, a bone-weakening disease that results from vitamin D deficiency, is becoming more common in this country. The small quantities of vitamin D in breast milk aren't enough unless your baby also spends some time in the sun, which stimulates the body to produce vitamin D. But since most parents keep their infants out of the sun to protect them against skin cancer, some infants are at risk for vitamin D deficiency and rickets. (Dark-skinned and African-American babies are most vulnerable because their skin needs more sunlight to produce vitamin D.)

As a result of these observations, the American Academy of Pediatrics is now recommending that breastfed infants receive 200 international units (IU)—or 5 milligrams—of vitamin D every day during the first 2 months of life and until they begin taking at least 15 ounces daily of vitamin D–fortified milk. This supplementation should be given in an over-the-counter liquid *multivitamin* preparation. (Vitamin D supplements alone are usually too concentrated to be safe for infants.)

The Academy also recommends a vitamin D supplement for infants who aren't breastfed and who don't drink at least 15 ounces of fortified formula or milk daily. Children and adolescents who consume less than that amount, who don't get regular sunlight exposure, or who don't take a multiple vitamin with at least 200 IU of vitamin D should also be given the vitamin D supplement.

THE BOTTOM LINE

Unless you have a good reason not to do so, you should breastfeed your infant. However, when your baby is at least 2 months old, add a daily multivitamin supplement containing 200 IU of vitamin D. This will protect against the possibility of rickets, the bone disease that can leave a child bowlegged and too short. Such supplementation also allows you to kept your child away from the harmful rays of the sun.

ROSACEA

· · · · · · · · ·

Improve Your First Impression

MANY PEOPLE DON'T KNOW much about rosacea, even though it affects 5 percent of Americans. Most assume it's due to alcoholism. My wife and I once attended a reception at Cornell University in honor of a man who had given the school a large amount of money. He was unpretentious, self-made, and of Irish ancestry. As we toasted our benefactor, someone whispered in my ear, "Isn't it amazing that such a boozer is so rich?"

"I didn't know he's a boozer," I said. "He certainly isn't drinking tonight."

The person replied, "Look at the guy's nose! You can practically see the alcohol oozing out of it." With a laugh, the amateur diagnostician downed the rest of his Scotch in one gulp and added, "It takes one to know one. He and I are both Irish."

My friend was right about our patron's Irish heritage, but he was wrong about the drinking. The guest of honor was, in fact, a teetotaler. Mistaking rosacea, a condition marked by a ruddy complexion and reddish nose (it can also appear on the neck, shoulders, chest, and back), for alcoholism is a common error. That is not to say that they can't coexist. Some of the 13 million people with rosacea probably do have a drinking problem, but the relationship is purely coincidental. The Irish connection, however, is real. A preponderance of rosacea patients in this country (39 percent in one survey) are of Celtic origin (Irish, Welsh, Highland Scottish), which is why this condition is sometimes referred to as the "curse of the Celts." However, people of English, eastern European, and Scandinavian ancestry are also prone to it.

Wrongfully tagging someone with rosacea as an alcoholic can be unfortunate both personally and professionally. In one survey of 400 people with this disorder, 35 percent stated that their skin condition was the reason they weren't hired in a new job or promoted in an old one; 70 percent said that they were embarrassed by their condition; 69 percent were frustrated by it; and 56 percent said rosacea had "robbed them of pleasure."

The cause of rosacea remains a mystery. Genetic factors may play a role since it occurs more often among the fair-skinned, and runs in families. All rosacea sufferers share one attribute—they blush easily. This may eventually dilate their blood vessels and leave a permanent facial discoloration. Although rosacea is more prevalent in women, it tends to be more severe in men. That may be because women pay more attention to their appearance than do men, see a doctor sooner about it, and so are treated early enough to slow the progression of their disease. Prompt therapy is important because half of rosacea patients develop ocular rosacea, or inflammation of the eye—the iris, conjunctiva, and even the cornea. (Corneal ulceration due to rosacea is a common cause of blindness.)

HERE'S WHAT'S NEW

There is no cure for rosacea, but the sooner you see a dermatologist about it, the better. Your symptoms can be improved; left untreated, they usually worsen.

If you have rosacea, anything that reddens your face will intensify the symptoms. The most common triggers, all of which you should avoid when possible, are as follows:

- Hot liquids
- Caffeine
- Sunlight (always use sunscreen with SPF of at least 30, preferably higher)
- Wind
- Hot and cold temperatures, including hot baths
- Spicy foods, especially white and black pepper, hot red peppers, paprika, cayenne, oriental mustard sauce, spicy nachos, or salsa
- Alcohol
- Stress and embarrassment (easier said than done)
- Overheating—after a strenuous workout or in a steam room (worsened by high humidity)
- The hot flashes of menopause

In addition to avoiding these triggers (and any others to which you are particularly sensitive), the following therapies will help:

- Terramycin (tetracycline) is the mainstay of treatment. I prefer two related antibiotics, Vibramycin (doxycycline) or Minocin (minocycline). They're easier on the gut than is Terramycin, and you don't have to take them on an empty stomach. If you can't tolerate this family of antibiotics, Erythrocin (erythromycin) is the next best choice.

• Topical Flagyl (metronidazole), is also sometimes given by mouth, is effective. In 1998 the FDA approved generic metronidazole topical therapy for rosacea. It is applied once a day.

• Topical steroids aggravate rosacea over the long term, but they may be used to reduce redness and irritation twice a day for a week or so.

• Avoid any topical preparations that contain alcohol, acetone, witch hazel, menthol, peppermint, eucalyptus oil, or clove oil.

• Make sure that whatever you put on your face has "noncomedogenic" written on the label. That means it does not clog pores.

• Use a daily skin moisturizer during cold weather to protect against the drying effects of cold and wind.

• Cover your cheeks and nose with a scarf when you go outdoors in winter, and wear a ski mask. (But remove it before going to your bank.)

• Men should use an electric razor rather than a blade, and don't apply any after-shave lotion that stings or burns.

• If you have heart disease, take the lowest possible dose of such vasodilator drugs as Isordil and Imdur (both forms of isosorbide) because they dilate blood vessels on your face as well as those in your heart.

• Niacin, which effectively lowers cholesterol, usually causes a flush and aggravates rosacea. Use a statin drug instead.

- Take clonidine if you blush easily. This is a potent blood-pressure-lowering drug, so check your pressure reading first.

- If and when dilated blood vessels become prominent and cosmetically embarrassing, they can be obliterated either by fine electric needles or by lasers.

THE BOTTOM LINE

The earlier you treat rosacea, the better. A dermatologist can prescribe the necessary antibiotics and topical medications that will minimize your symptoms.

SEXUAL
DYSFUNCTION

· · · · · · · · ·

When Viagra Doesn't Work

IN ORDER TO ENSURE a satisfactory erection, the penis must receive enough blood. Viagra (sildenafil) has helped improve bloodflow for many men with erectile dysfunction, as evidenced by the 20 million prescriptions for it and the estimated one billion pills consumed. But bloodflow is not the only factor necessary for producing an erection. Men also must produce enough testosterone—the hormone that gives us both libido *and* an erection. (It also helps prevent osteoporosis, depression, and fatigue.) Between four million and five million men are believed to be testosterone deficient. So the following news should be of great interest to them.

HERE'S WHAT'S NEW

Viagra works by making more nitric oxide available to the penis. This chemical relaxes the smooth muscles in the penis and widens its arteries, thus providing the extra blood needed for an erection. Researchers at New York's Columbia Presbyterian Medical Center have found that nitric oxide requires testosterone in order to function properly. When a man is deficient in this hormone, the nitric oxide released by Viagra may not work. They suggest that in such cases, Viagra's potency can be restored by supplemental testosterone delivered through the skin in a gel.

THE BOTTOM LINE

As a man ages, his testosterone level decreases. This is a gradual, normal, and natural phenomenon that usually does not cause symptoms. A man of 80 has much less testosterone than one of 30 but can still produce enough sperm to father a child. However, testosterone levels can and often do become low enough to cause several symptoms (some call it "male menopause"), among them impotence.

If you have erectile dysfunction, get a complete medical exam, including a testosterone level test. If your your hormone level is low, ask your doctor about replacing it. If that does not restore potency, then add Viagra.

Viagra after Prostate Surgery

MEN WITH PROSTATE CANCER have several treatment options, depending on their age, their health, and the stage of their disease. Younger patients who are better operative risks usually choose surgery. Beyond the age of 65 or 70, some form of radiation (either external or from implanted seeds) is preferred. Older men or those in whom the disease has spread and is no longer curable by surgery or radiation are treated with various hormones. Some whose tumors are not particularly aggressive may opt for "watchful waiting" (their condition is closely followed for evidence of progression). Every one of these treatments, with the exception of the last, carries with it some side effects, most of which are troublesome but manageable.

It used to be that surgical treatment of prostate cancer almost always resulted in impotence and urinary incontinence. These complications have been somewhat reduced, but by no means eliminated, since the development of a "nerve-sparing" operation by Patrick Walsh, M.D., at Johns Hopkins University School of Medicine in Baltimore.

HERE'S WHAT'S NEW

Researchers at the University of California, Los Angeles, have confirmed the effectiveness of Viagra in treating impotence resulting from prostate cancer surgery. However, they have found it to be more effective when used in a different way. Instead of taking the 50- or 100-milligram tablet 1 hour before planned sexual relations, they recommend that patients should take it regularly every night for 9 months after their operation—whether or not they're having (or trying to have) sex.

After 9 months, men so treated were seven times more likely to be as potent as they were before their operation than were those unfortunate enough to have fallen into the placebo category (a risk you always take when you sign up for a double-blind study!). Twenty-seven percent of the Viagra-treated patients regained normal erectile function, compared with only 4 percent of the placebo receivers.

Why not just give these men the Viagra tablet whenever they plan to have sex? Why the nightly dosing for 9 months (during which time sex may not always be on their mind)? The researchers believe that the 9-month treatment may *prevent* impotence and eliminate the need for pill-by-pill Viagra later on. They suggest that Viagra facilitates an erection in such cases not only by increasing blood flow to the penis but also by repairing nerve damage sustained during the operation. They consider their findings to be so dramatic that they are recommending this 9-month Viagra therapy for every man who has had a prostatectomy for whatever reason and who is interested in having sex in the future.

Incidentally, Viagra has stiff competition from two chemically related drugs, Cialis (tadalafil) and Levitra (vardenafil).

THE BOTTOM LINE

Sexually active men who have had a radical prostatectomy should consider taking a daily Viagra tablet for 9 months after surgery to increase their chances of resuming normal sexual function in the future. Bear in mind, however, that people with heart disease who are taking nitroglycerin-type drugs or other blood pressure–lowering agents such as alpha-blockers Hytrin (terazosin) and Cardura (doxazosin) should use Viagra with caution. The combinating can cause a dangerous drop in blood pressure.

Multiple Viagra Benefits for Women

WHEN A WOMAN'S ESTROGEN LEVELS are markedly reduced, such as happens with menopause or after a total hysterectomy, she may lose interest in sex or derive little pleasure from it. For a woman motivated to do something about it, the usual treatment initially is estrogen supplementation. If that doesn't help, small doses of testosterone are often prescribed and are more effective.

Because of the impact of Viagra on male erectile dysfunction, it has been suggested that this drug can also enhance sexual pleasure in women, presumably by increasing blood flow to sensitive areas in the female genitalia, including the clitoris.

HERE'S WHAT'S NEW

Researchers at the Female Sexual Medicine Center at UCLA in Los Angeles and Northwestern University in Chicago have made some preliminary observations about Viagra's effect on female sexual satisfaction after a double-blind study of 202 postmenopausal or posthysterectomy women who complained of diminished libido. The treated group received either a 50- or 100-milligram Viagra tablet prior to sexual activity, no more than once a day. They were screened to exclude the possibility that psychological or relationship issues might account for their problems. The participants were asked to keep notes of their reactions after every sex experience. (Now you know what your wife was busily writing the last time you were intimate.)

The Viagra-treated group reported a significantly higher incidence of orgasms than did those who received placebos. Some experienced the same mild side effects of which some men complain, namely flushing, headache, nausea, and visual symptoms.

The doctors conducting the study believe that this orgasmic response was the result of increased blood flow to the female genitals, with better arousal, sensation, and lubrication.

It is estimated that some 43 percent of women aren't very interested in sex or derive little pleasure from it—and they are not all menopausal. In many cases, it's the result of an unsatisfactory emotional relationship—and Viagra is not likely to help that. It's for that reason that Pfizer, the maker of Viagra, has stopped its research on

Viagra for women. They believe that the major factors in women's sexual dissatisfaction are psychological rather than physical. However, there is a subset of women in whom Viagra can increase the joy of sex, regardless of their hormonal status. I'm referring to those being treated for depression. One of the side effects of the most commonly used antidepressants, including Prozac (fluoxetine) and Zoloft (sertraline), is "sexual dysfunction."

Recent research results published in the *Journal of the American Medical Association* indicate that among depressed *men* on these drugs whose libido was significantly reduced, the addition of Viagra increased arousal or sexual satisfaction. The same researchers found similar results in women and presented them at the 51st annual meeting of the American College of Obstetricians and Gynecologists. They suggest that Viagra be taken at the start of the antidepressant therapy so as to prevent the decrease in libido that sometimes leads women to discontinue their therapy.

THE BOTTOM LINE

If your sexual pleasure is noticeably diminished after menopause or a hysterectomy, you'll likely be advised to take some form of hormone replacement. Assuming you have no other significant symptoms due to hormone depletion, in view of all the discussion about the adverse effects of its long-term replacement therapy, you may want to consider trying Viagra first. There's no downside to it. The same is true for women of any age who have been treated with antidepressant drugs that interfered with their libidos.

If it turns out that Viagra doesn't work for you, you'll be happy to know that the money you spent on the Viagra was not wasted. Adding a small piece of a Viagra pill to the water in a vase may keep your flowers from wilting! Two scientists had previously found that nitric oxide extends the shelf life of fruits and vegetables. Viagra, like nitric oxide, inhibits the enzyme that breaks down energy-rich molecules in plants. In so doing, it keeps flowers erect and alive for up to 7 days longer. These findings were presented at an International Conference on Fresh-Cut Produce in England.

My wife has tried Viagra—on her flowers—and she tells me it works. But I haven't yet read any comments about this use from Pfizer, the maker of Viagra.

SEXUALLY
TRANSMITTED
DISEASES

* * * * * * * * * *

A Sad State of Affairs

THE TERM "SEXUALLY TRANSMITTED DISEASE" (STD) refers to any infection—bacterial, viral, or parasitic—that is transmitted primarily by sexual contact. Although the entry sites are most commonly oral, vaginal, penile, or anal, organisms can penetrate the body through a nonsexual route such as a cut or sore in the skin, and babies can be infected during birth. One of every four people worldwide will one day contract a sexually transmitted disease. Aside from AIDS, an estimated 56 million Americans already harbor at least one such infection, and millions more are newly infected every year.

Despite increasing public education, the incidence of some STDs continues to rise. Here's where we currently stand with the most important of these infections.

Chlamydia. Many millions of men and women have chlamydia in addition to the more who contract it every year making it the most common STD in the United States. Chlamydia caused by a bacterium called *Chlamydia trachomatis* that is transmitted during unprotected vaginal or anal sex. Any one of a number of antibiotics can cure chlamydia easily. The problem is that it causes no symptoms in 70 percent of women and 30 percent of men infected who are unaware they have it, and continue to infect their sexual partners. By the time they discover it, females may have developed pelvic inflammatory disease with chronic, severe pelvic pain, have a 20 percent chance of infertility, and a 10 percent likelihood of having an ectopic pregnancy (because the chlamydia bug scars the fallopian tubes). If a woman with untreated chlamydia does retain her pregnancy, her baby may be born prematurely, have a low birth weight, and/or develop pneumonia or conjunctivitis (a threat to vision later in life). Men with chronic chlamydia may develop chronic infection of the urethra and swollen, tender testicles. Left untreated, they become infertile.

Symptoms of chlamydia infection, when they do occur, appear anywhere from 1 to 3 weeks after exposure. Women usually have a yellowish-green vaginal discharge or vaginal bleeding, painful urination, pain and bleeding during intercourse, and chronic lower abdominal pain; men may develop a burning sensation when they urinate and a whitish mucoid discharge from the penis. The *Chlamydia* bacterium can cause an inflamed rectum and a sore throat from anal and oral sex.

Gonorrhea. Although the incidence of gonorrhea has been declining over the years, there are still over one million new cases reported annually. (Imagine how many remain in the closet.) This disease is easy to treat but doesn't always cause symptoms. I've known men who would go to the nearest emergency room after a sexual fling for a shot of penicillin just in case. That doesn't always work anymore, because many strains of gonorrhea have become resistant to penicillin. However, a wide range of antibiotics still eradicate this infection.

Gonorrhea is caused by a bacterium called *Neisseria gonorrhoeae*, which is spread by unprotected oral, vaginal, or anal sex. Gonorrhea is the only STD that can be transmitted by "eye contact." If you scratch your infected genitals and then rub your eye, you may develop ocular gonorrhea, which can lead to blindness if untreated. Pregnant women also can transmit the infection to their babies.

Gonorrhea is not apparent in most infected women and in 20 percent of infected men. When symptoms do appear in men, anywhere from 1 day to 2 weeks after exposure, they consist of a discharge of yellowish pus from the tip of the penis accompanied by burning and stinging during urination. Blood may be visible in the urine, the head of the penis may be inflamed and red, and the glands in the groin may swell. Women develop a cloudy vaginal discharge, irritation of the external genitalia, burning on urination, and irregular menstrual bleeding.

If untreated, women eventually end up with pelvic inflammatory disease involving the fallopian tubes, uterus, and ovaries. Men can develop chronic infection of the prostate gland and testicles, as well as a septic form of arthritis of the knee or the elbow.

Syphilis. There are 120,000 new cases of syphilis are reported every year. It remains a treacherous infection because you may not know you have it and so can unwittingly spread it.

Primary syphilis begins as a painless sore at the site of infection (the sex organs or the mouth) that is easily mistaken for a harmless cold sore. After this initial warning, the *Treponema pallidum* bacterium that causes syphilis goes into hiding for weeks or months. When it does reappear, it causes a rash anywhere in the body (secondary syphilis). If you don't think of syphilis at this stage and are not treated, the third stage is next. It may not appear for years, but when it does, it can kill or cripple you, striking anywhere—the heart, the brain, or any other vital organ. Syphilis is easily diagnosed with a simple blood test. All three stages are treated with penicillin—the earlier, the better.

Genital herpes. Genital herpes is so benign an infection when compared to the other STDs that most people don't take it seriously anymore, despite the 40 million who have its chronic form and the 500,000 new cases that occur each year.

But it's a mistake to ignore herpes. Its sores not only are painful and annoying, but can also create serious problems to a newborn who contracts it at birth (see page 337). The infection is caused by one of two viruses, herpes simplex virus (HSV) 1 or 2, mostly the latter. As with other STDs, you may be infected and never know it, or you may develop painful bumps and sores at the site of infection days or weeks after exposure. You can get herpes not only from oral, anal, or genital sex but also by touching someone's sore with a break in your skin, or by kissing. The infection can flare up or recur at any time and there is no cure for it. You can catch it or transmit it even when there are no visible lesions. Zovirax (acyclovir) and several other newer antiviral agents have made a big difference in the lives of those infected with herpes. These medications shorten the duration of the outbreaks, reduce their severity when taken early enough, and also delay or prevent recurrences.

HPV. The human papilloma virus (HPV) that causes genital warts infects some 40 million American men and women, whose ranks are joined by 1 million new cases every year. Thirteen of the more than

70 types of HPV are present in virtually every case of cervical cancer and are presumed to cause it.

HPV causes a variety of warts in the genital and anal areas that may appear as soft, pink, cauliflower-shaped lesions or hard, smooth, yellow-gray ones. This virus attacks both men and women. The wart may be hard to find if it is hidden inside the folds of the vagina. When HPV affects the cervix, it can cause to cervical cancer. Although there are several treatments for the warts (lasers, freezing, burning), the infection itself cannot be cured and the warts may reappear at any time.

Hepatitis B. Hepatitis B is a viral infection of the liver that strikes at least 300,000 Americans every year. The B virus is 100 times more infectious than the HIV that causes AIDS; both are spread primarily through infected blood. But there is one big difference: A vaccine can protect you from hepatitis B; there is no vaccine for AIDS yet. I recommend vaccination to most of my patients, and I insist on it for those who are healthcare workers or who are vulnerable because of their sexual lifestyle. There is no treatment for acute hepatitis B other than rest. However, the chronic form that causes liver cirrhosis and cancer in some patients may respond to interferon (see page 193).

Trichomoniasis. "Trich" is a common, non-life-threatening STD caused by a protozoan organism called *Trichomonas vaginalis*. There are 2 million to 3 million new cases every year. Many of those infected have no symptoms; others experience burning on urination, vaginal discharge, abdominal pain, or painful intercourse. Both sex partners should be treated, even if only one is known to be infected. A single dose of Flagyl (metronidazole) will often cure the infection.

HIV/AIDS. One million Americans are currently infected by the killer HIV/AIDS virus, which strikes an additional 40,000 people in the United States every year. It's the deadliest of all the STDs and there is currently no cure for it. Most of those infected eventually die as a result of the failure of their immune system, which is attacked and compromised by the HIV virus. Symptoms of AIDS may not appear until months or years after infection, during which time the disease is progressing. There are many new treatments that can delay death and improve the quality of life. If you test positive for HIV, consult a specialist to decide when the drugs, notably the protease inhibitors, should be started.

HERE'S WHAT'S NEW

The newest breakthroughs in STD treatment and prevention can benefit those with herpes or HIV/AIDS (see pages 337 and 333). Meanwhile, the basics of STD prevention and treatment are worth reviewing since many people still don't understand them (as evidenced by the growing rate of infection). Remember that many sexually transmitted diseases exist together; infection with one means that you might have others. The diagnosis of any STD makes it imperative to search for the others, especially HIV.

STD prevention boils down to *everyone* practicing safe sex—heterosexuals, homosexuals, men and women of all ages, of every background, and all income groups. Because of their anatomy, women are more likely to become infected during unprotected sex than are men, but no one is immune. The only prevention that's 100 percent effective is total abstinence; your next best bet is *always* to use a condom—not just once in a while or when you think there is some risk, but every time you indulge—unless you and your partner are monogamous and not infected.

STDs can be transmitted in ways other than vaginal and anal sex, notably by kissing, touching, and sharing needles. Condoms won't protect you in those situations.

All pregnant women should be tested for syphilis and hepatitis. Those who test positive should work with their doctors to protect their infants. If there's any question of exposure, pregnant women should also be tested for gonorrhea, have a Pap test, and be offered an HIV exam. Some doctors recommend that women with recurrent genital herpes with sores have a cesarean section in order to protect their unborn child.

If you're hooked on drugs, remember that it's dangerous to share needles. Ask about rehabilitation programs in your area that provide clean needles. If there is *any* possibility that you were infected in a relationship, inform your doctor and tell *all* your sex partners too.

THE BOTTOM LINE

STDs are more common and easier to contract than most people think. The sooner an infection is diagnosed, the greater the chances of curing it. Don't wait for symptoms; they may take a long time to show up. Even the tests for STD may not become positive until weeks after exposure.

A Breakthrough Drug for AIDS

AIDS IS THE MODERN-DAY PLAGUE. Most afflicted are men between ages 25 and 44. The greatest problem is in sub-Saharan Africa, where more than one in four people are infected. Tragically, many cannot afford therapy and millions will die in the next few years.

Although there is no cure for AIDS, drugs are available that can slow its progress and improve the quality of the years a person has left. Antiretroviral drugs that attack HIV and interfere with its ability to reproduce in the body, fall into three main groups that yield the best results when used together. All three categories work by neutralizing one or more of the enzymes that the virus needs in order to multiply. When combined, they attack three or four enzymes simultaneously and paralyze the virus at least temporarily.

Unfortunately, even the most effective combination of antiretrovirals does not eradicate the virus from the bloodstream. It simply moves to another area of the body or continues to replicate at a much slower rate. Still, patients do feel better when they take these drugs and can often resume a near-normal life, occasionally years.

The downside to these drugs is that they are potentially toxic, and are eventually abondoned by as many as half the patients taking them because of their intolerable side effects. They are also expensive and their dosage schedules are inconvenient.

One group of antiretrovirals is nucleoside reverse transcriptase inhibitors, which block the crucial viral enzyme reverse transcriptase. This particular drug is used alone only in pregnant women to prevent transmission of the virus to the infant.

Protease inhibitors are the second group of antiretrovirals. They suppress the viral enzyme protease. The third, and most recent addition to the anti-AIDS armamentarium, is the nonnucleoside reverse transcriptase inhibitors. They inhibit the same enzyme as does the nucleoside group, but in a different way.

HERE'S WHAT'S NEW

The FDA recently approved Fuzeon (enfuvirtide), a major medical advance representing a totally new class of AIDS drugs called fusion inhibitors. They fight advanced HIV when all other treatments fail. This new therapy is especially welcome in patients who are resistant to earlier treatments.

Here's what's new about Fuzeon: Whereas the older drugs acted on the HIV *after* it had infected the human cells and prevented the virus from replicating, Fuzeon stops HIV from getting into the cells in the first place. Unfortunately, Fuzeon is not easy to take and it's expensive, requiring two daily injections and costing more than $20,000 a year. It can also have serious side effects, such as pneumonia.

THE BOTTOM LINE

If you have AIDS, the right drug can improve the quality of your life and prolong it. There are several drugs available that are quite effective. However, when they have stopped working, speak to your doctor (and your health insurance carrier) about Fuzeon, a new drug that can make a big difference.

Get HIV Test Results in 3 to 20 Minutes

ALMOST ONE MILLION AMERICANS are HIV positive or live with AIDS. According to the Centers for Disease Control and Prevention, as many as one-third of them are unaware that they have it, so it's vital that you get tested if you think you may have been exposed to the virus.

Until recently, patients typically had to wait at least a week for the results of blood tests for HIV that were sent to a laboratory. The mounting anxiety as well as a natural tendency for denial resulted each year in an estimated 8,000 infected people simply not coming back to learn their test results.

HERE'S WHAT'S NEW

The FDA has approved two rapid HIV tests that require only a drop of blood from your finger. Although the first, OraQuick, was originally available only to laboratories, it is now used in doctors' offices and HIV counseling centers. It is 99.6 percent accurate and provides results in about 20 minutes. The second test, the Reveal Rapid HIV-1 Antibody Test kit, gives the answer in 3 minutes. However, it's designed for use only in hospitals and clinics.

But wait! You ain't heard nothin' yet. The latest news is there is yet a third way to test for HIV—in the privacy of your own home. You get the result in about a minute! All it requires is one drop of blood obtained from a fingerstick. Simply add the blood to a blue filter and look for the color change. This "One-Minute Self Test" is sold in Monaco and 30 other countries, but not yet in the United States. The manufacturer states that it is more than 99 percent accurate and meets or exceeds the sensitivity and specificity of available FDA-approved tests. Look for its release in this country.

These new tests also make it possible for health care workers who have been accidentally exposed to infected blood to learn sooner whether they contracted the virus that causes AIDS. Pregnant women going into labor who are tested and found to be HIV-positive can now be treated in time to prevent transmitting the disease to their newborns. And if you're worried about having contracted the disease, you won't have to wait a week or longer for an answer. These tests cost about $40, and there is no public record of the results since only you and your doctor are privy to them.

THE BOTTOM LINE

If you think you may have been exposed to HIV, you can now ask your doctor or an HIV-counseling clinic to draw a drop of blood from your finger, test it for this infection, and give you the results then and there. No more sleepless nights waiting for an answer and fearing the worst—often unnecessarily. Even though a 1-minute, home-testing kit is available in Europe, I suggest that, for the time being, you use the two varieties sold in this country.

Protect Your Newborn from Herpes

THE HERPES SIMPLEX VIRUS (HSV) used to be of major concern to millions of Americans. However, the HIV/AIDS epidemic has taken center stage among the sexually transmitted diseases, and HSV is much less on our minds these days. What's more, the availability of new antiviral agents, such as Zovirax (acyclovir) and Famvir (famciclovir), has reduced both the recurrence rate of herpetic sores and the likelihood of transmission to an uninfected partner.

Although herpes is not as much of a threat as other sexually transmitted diseases such as human papillomavirus (which can lead to cervical cancer), it's still unpleasant and embarrassing. As the old Packard advertising slogan put it, just "ask the man (or woman) who owns one!"

When the virus is transmitted to a newborn, it can cause brain damage or even death. This is especially likely to happen if the mother recently acquired herpes (her immune system has not yet been able to make antibodies to the virus, that could then be passed to her child).

HERE'S WHAT'S NEW

It has long been suspected but never really proven that delivery by Cesarean section in women with active herpes significantly reduces the risk of infecting their newborns. Recent research has shown this to be a fact. In a study of some 200 pregnant women with herpes, only 1 percent of those who underwent Cesarean section gave birth to children with HSV, compared with the nearly 8 percent who delivered vaginally.

THE BOTTOM LINE

Obstetricians suggest that every pregnant woman be screened for genital herpes at her first prenatal care visit. If the test result is positive, she should be treated with one of the antiviral drugs mentioned above. If she was recently infected, she should consider having a Cesarean delivery, especially if she has genital sores.

It's also a good idea for the father to be checked, too. If the mother tests negative but her partner is harboring the virus, he should take an antiviral drug at least during the entire pregnancy. He should always use a condom or abstain from sex until after the baby is born, in order not to infect the mother and her child.

SHINGLES

• • • • • • • • •

Act Fast for Best Results

VIRUSES ARE LIKE the man who came to dinner. They are uninvited and outstay their welcome. One of the worst viral offenders is the varicella-zoster virus (VZV), which causes chickenpox. After it attacks little children, covering them with harmful sores and making them miserable for days, it migrates to the nerve centers along the spine, where it takes up permanent residence, only to reappear years later making its victims miserable when they're adults.

In most cases, VZV remains reclusive and dormant in its "retirement." However, in about 20 percent of its hosts, it "wakes up." Ungrateful for the hospitality that its victim has provided over the years, it retraces its steps along the nerve pathways it ascended years ago and once again, causes pain and blisters on the skin. This time, however, with an even greater vengeance. We don't call this illness chickenpox. The second time around it's *shingles*.

The hallmark of shingles is that without having hurt yourself, you develop burning or shooting pain, or numbness, tingling, or itching, in some part of your body—the trunk, back, chest, face, spine, neck, near an eye or an ear—but *only on one side*. It may be proceded by flu-like symptoms such as headache, fever, chills, and nausea followed a few days later by the appearance of a telltale red, painful rash where you felt the original symptoms. If the shingles virus affects one of your eyes, see an ophthalmologist immediately. Ocular shingles can end in blindness.

Until recent years, treatment of shingles consisted of little more than ointments and painkillers. However, antiviral drugs have changed the course of this illness. Doctors can now better relieve the agony of post-herpetic neuralgia (PHN)—the most dreaded complication of shingles which severe pain persists for months and occasionally years after the rash and other symptoms have disappeared. PHN develops in about 15 percent of patients overall (more than 50 percent of whom are over age 60).

There are several effective antivirals for shingles. Although the oldest, Zovirax (acyclovir), still works, the newer Famvir (famciclovir) and Valtrex (valacyclovir) have a better track record in reducing the chances of your developing post-herpetic neuralgia.

Once you have PHN, it's too late for antivirals; you now need painkillers. First, try one of the non-prescription nonsteroidal anti-inflammatory drugs (NSAIDs), such as Advil (ibuprofen). Or ask your doctor to prescribe Elavil (amitriptyline), a tricyclic antidepressant that works by blocking serotonin and adrenaline uptake in the brain, or apply a local anesthetic such as the topical Lidoderm (lidocaine) patch.

To reduce your chances of getting shingles, have the chickenpox (varicella) vaccine if you've never had chickenpox. And get your kids vaccinated, too. This virus has been plaguing mankind since time immemorial, but its heady, carefree days may be numbered. The new safe and effective vaccine against chickenpox means that more kids may become immune to and never get this infection—or shingles!

HERE'S WHAT'S NEW

The introduction of specific antiviral drugs has changed the course of shingles and the long-term complications. These agents don't kill the virus, but they prevent it from reproducing by inhibiting one of its DNA enzymes. By doing so they lessen pain, shorten the duration of symptoms, and dramatically reduce the risk of PHN if you take them within 72 hours after symptoms start. The shocking fact is that fewer than 50 percent of patients with shingles see a doctor within this optimal window of opportunity. You must recognize the symptoms of the disease and be aware that the sooner you get treatment, the better off you'll be.

THE BOTTOM LINE

The moment you know (or have good reason to suspect) that you have shingles, see your doctor right away. Unless you start treatment with one of the newer antivirals within 72 hours, you may be in for prolonged pain and suffering due to PHN.

SINUSITIS

. . . .

Curing Chronic Sinus Infection

IT'S NEITHER LIFE-THREATENING NOR CONTAGIOUS, but chronic sinusitis is a real pain—in the head. The postnasal drip and constant
throat clearing, chronic cough, recurrent headache, nasal congestion,
and tenderness around the eyes and cheeks can make you miserable
for months.

Sinusitis is an infection and inflammation of the sinus cavities in
the face and head caused by viruses or bacteria. Allergic individuals
whose mucous membranes are chronically irritated and swollen are
sitting ducks for such infection. Sinusitis is difficult to cure because
antibiotics can't easily penetrate the closed sinus spaces. The usual
scenario is round after round of antibiotics in the hope that a new
and different one will solve the problem. It rarely does—for any

length of time. Some patients require surgery to drain the infected sinuses.

HERE'S WHAT'S NEW

Researchers at Stanford University in California have successfully treated chronic sinusitis by delivering the antibiotics via a nasal mist rather than orally or by injection. They prescribed these inhaled antibiotics for 3 weeks to 42 adults whose sinusitis persisted, even after surgical drainage, and who were on the verge of being given intravenous antibiotics. The nasal mist eliminated the infection in 76 percent of cases for at least 3 months after the treatment ended. The results were published in the journal *Otolaryngology—Head and Neck Surgery*.

THE BOTTOM LINE

If you suffer from chronic sinusitis that keeps coming back, ask your doctor about getting the antibiotic via a nasal mist. It's something you can do yourself, and it may cure the infection more effectively than oral medication.

SMALLPOX

●●●●●●●●●

When *Not* to Be Vaccinated

I REMEMBER how happy I was several years ago to read that smallpox was no more, that it had been eradicated forever. What a triumph for science and public health! Unfortunately, mankind was not civilized enough to take advantage of the demise of this killer agent. We (yes, that includes our own country) decided it would be wise to keep some of this lethal virus alive in a "secure location" just in case we ever needed to kill an enemy sometime, somewhere down the line. There was no public referendum on the matter—just a political-military decision. So we stockpiled smallpox virus, as did our then enemies, the Russians. Even after the end of the Cold War, both nations held onto their smallpox supplies. As they say in the New York lotto, "Hey, you never know." The world's leaders must have decided that our arsenal of nuclear weapons and other horrendous instruments of mass destruction, both biological and biochemical—viruses, gases, and poisons—were not enough.

Now, years later, we're forced once more to think about protecting ourselves against this terrible disease, not because it has reappeared in nature, but in the event that some rogue state or terrorist group decides to attack us with it. Our own smallpox arsenal is said to be secure and intact, but we cannot vouch for any deadly germs that others have. The possibility of the theft or sale of live smallpox virus is real enough to constitute a threat to our allies and to us.

The last routine smallpox vaccination was administered in this country in the early 1970s, and presumably anyone who received it then is no longer fully protected. As a result, our government has made vaccination mandatory for the military. (George W. Bush already has had his shot.) It is recommended, but not required, for health care professionals who may be called upon to treat victims of an attack. The vaccine is optional for the rest of the population. Whether you choose to have it depends on how real you perceive the threat to be. However, anyone who has been directly exposed to the virus must take the vaccine because the disease itself is much more dangerous than the consequences of the vaccine.

Given the renewed and widespread interest in (and fear of) smallpox, together with the fact that many people will be opting to take the vaccine, the Centers for Disease Control and Prevention (CDC) has recently updated its advice about who should *not* be getting it. *Do not take the vaccine if you're known to be allergic to it or if any of the following apply to you:*

Eczema or atopic dermatitis. Even if you had this skin problem years ago as a child, it places you at high risk for various serious, occasionally fatal skin reactions as well as encephalitis.

Other skin conditions. Any acute, chronic, or peeling skin disorder, including a burn, impetigo, chickenpox, shingles, contact dermatitis, herpes, severe acne, diaper rash, or psoriasis. Wait until the condition has completely cleared before being vaccinated.

Darier's disease. A rare genetic skin disorder.

A compromised immune system. The smallpox vaccine contains a live virus called vaccinia. It isn't the smallpox virus itself, but it's so closely related to it that it stimulates the same protective antibody response. Anything that suppresses your immune system leaves you vulnerable to unchecked spread of the live vaccinia virus within your body, but primarily on your skin. That includes conditions such as HIV/AIDS, any organ transplant (but not artificial joints such as knees or hips), any type of malignancy, or lupus. Chemotherapy and steroid hormones can also leave you immunosuppressed.

Moderate or severe acute illness. It isn't a good idea to be vaccinated if you're in the throes of the flu, pneumonia, or any other illness or infection. Wait until you've recovered from it.

Pregnancy and breastfeeding. Any live-virus vaccination is inadvisable during pregnancy, and smallpox is no exception. Although uncommon, the risk of an adverse reaction affecting the fetus is real. Also do not receive the vaccine while you're breastfeeding because it's not known whether the virus is transmitted through breast milk.

Infants and children. Infants younger than age 12 months should not be vaccinated against smallpox, and the vaccine is not recommended to those younger than age 18 (excluding military personnel), except in an emergency.

Do not receive the vaccine if anyone in your household is also vulnerable to its complications because when you are vaccinated, you can transmit the vaccinia virus (but not smallpox) to them if they come in contact with the vaccination site or with clothing or material that has been in contact with it.

Although doctors have been made aware of these contraindications, they are still "new" to most of us because we have not been thinking about smallpox for more than 30 years.

HERE'S WHAT'S NEW

The current vaccination program was formulated on the assumption that immunity from smallpox vaccine lasts only 5 years. However, researchers now believe that this immunity lasts much longer. This new information is based on tests of people who were vaccinated as long as 75 years ago. Every one of them was found to have some immunity to the smallpox virus. In more than 90 percent of them, the level of antibodies was high enough to prevent serious infection. That would argue against the need for mass vaccination, and support limiting vaccination to health workers, the military, and others at especially high risk.

The roughly 120 million people born since 1972, when the last shot was given in this country, obviously have no immunity to smallpox. But if you're older than age 35, and did receive the vaccine at least once, there's a 90 percent chance you probably are still protected. That's big news, and it should help you decide whether or not to be vaccinated again now.

Since the current vaccination program went into effect, there have been 17 cardiac events, 3 of them fatal, associated with the vaccine among the 30,000 civilians and 300,000 military personnel who received it. Most occurred in individuals with previous evidence of heart trouble, such as angina. Although a cause and effect relationship has not been established definitively, the CDC is recommending that anyone with an existing heart problem not be given the vaccine. Doctors postulate that the vaccine results in generalized inflammation that may aggravate an underlying cardiac disorder.

THE BOTTOM LINE

It's up to you whether or not to take the smallpox vaccine. However, if your immune system is weakened for any reason, or you have a heart condition or one of the skin disorders described, do not be vaccinated. Remember that this applies if anyone in your household is susceptible to the vaccine's adverse effects because when you take the vaccine, you become a "carrier" as far as they are concerned.

I am recommending it only for those patients who are health care workers or who are likely to be in close contact with an infected individual in the event of a terrorist attack. I do not plan to take it myself because I am counting on the immunity conferred by my last shot some 35 years ago.

Having said all that, let me emphasize two key points. First, if you choose not to have the vaccine at this time for any reason and terrorists attack with the virus, there is a window of about 4 days after exposure during which vaccination protect you. Second, even if you have any condition that precludes being vaccinated now in the event of a *future* attack, you will have to be vaccinated if and when such an attack occurs.

Donating Blood after Vaccination

THE GOVERNMENT HAS RECOMMENDED that some Americans be vaccinated against smallpox because of a possible terror attack. Many individuals at greatest risk (health care providers and military personnel) have already received the vaccine that contains the live virus. For the moment, smallpox vaccination remains optional for the rest of the population and is not recommended at this time because its risks may outweigh its benefits.

HERE'S WHAT'S NEW

If you recently have been vaccinated and are thinking of donating blood, you must take certain precautions because the vaccine you were given contains a live virus that can be transmitted to anyone who receives your blood. So don't donate (other than to yourself) for at least 3 weeks after getting the shot or until the scab at the injection site falls off, whichever is later. If you had an adverse reaction to the vaccine, delay giving blood for at least 14 days after that reaction has cleared up. If you aren't asked about smallpox vaccination at the blood bank, be sure to volunteer this information.

THE BOTTOM LINE

Hold off on donating your blood for at least 3 weeks after being vaccinated for smallpox, because the live vaccine it contains can be transmitted to who may not be able to tolerate it.

STROKE

. . . .

Prevention: Something Old, Something New

Despite all the new sophisticated technology to diagnose whatever ails you, the old-fashioned stethoscope remains an important tool. Unfortunately, doctors use it less and less these days. They either leave it in a coat pocket with just enough showing as their "ID" or, what's even more chic, they drape it around the neck. Who needs a necktie with such professional attire?

Besides using the stethoscope to examine your heart and lungs, it's important for your doctor to place it over the arteries in your neck to listen for a *bruit* (pronounced *broo-ee*). This is the sound generated by blood flowing through a narrowed artery, in this case the carotids that carry the blood from the heart through the neck into the brain. When one or both of these arteries are significantly narrowed, you are at risk for having a stroke. What a simple, inexpensive way to detect a life-threatening condition!

If your doctor hears a bruit, the next step is a carotid sonogram. That's also simple to do, but a lot more expensive. It determines the degree of blockage so that you and your doctor can decide whether anything needs to be done about it. The loudness of the bruit does not always reflect the severity of the obstruction. In other words, a soft sound may reflect a serious problem and a loud one may not. However, *every bruit requires evaluation.*

If the obstruction is found to be "high grade"—that is, severe enough to warrant removal—there are two ways to do so. The first is called a carotid endarterectomy, in which the obstructing plaque in the arterial wall is surgically scraped away. In a newer, nonsurgical technique, the artery is ballooned open and then kept open with a sleeve called a stent. This is similar to the technique used to treat diseased coronary arteries in the heart.

HERE'S WHAT'S NEW

Doctors have been compiling statistics to compare the safety and efficacy of surgery and stenting of carotid artery blockages. The results are now in. Stenting wins hands down as the procedure of choice for patients at high risk. What has made the difference is the use of an ingenious little "umbrella" (called an AngioGuard) that's inserted into the neck artery before the stenting procedure. It traps any debris or little pieces of the plaques that may break off during the procedure, so they don't travel up to the brain and cause a stroke. After the stenting is finished, the umbrella is removed.

This combination of stent and the AngioGuard has reduced many of the complications of surgery in carotid artery obstruction in high-risk patients. Here's how results with both techniques compare:

Thirty days after each procedure, the rate of stroke, heart attack, or death in the stented group was 5.8 percent; in those treated surgically, it was 12.6 percent. As far as strokes alone are concerned, the incidence in stented patients was 3.8 percent; in the surgical group, 5.3 percent. The risk of heart attacks was 2.6 percent versus 7.3 percent. So stenting is safer in every respect.

THE BOTTOM LINE

Always make sure your doctor listens carefully to your neck during a routine physical examination. Carotid blockages usually don't cause symptoms—your doctor must listen for them. If he or she hears an abnormal sound (a bruit), you should be further tested with a carotid sonogram. If that reveals a blockage severe enough to require correcting, ask your doctor how it will be done. If the answer is surgical endarterectomy, ask about the stenting procedure. It may not be offered as an option because it's relatively new and not done in every hospital.

Can You Recognize the Signs of a Stroke?

IT'S INCREDIBLE BUT TRUE: Most people having a stroke, even when it's severe enough to send them to a hospital, don't know the cause of their illness. This is also true of bystanders and family members. Stroke education is important because interpreting the symptoms quickly and getting to the hospital as soon as possible permits early treatment that can reduce the long-term complications of this "cerebrovascular accident."

HERE'S WHAT'S NEW

Researchers at the University of North Carolina in Chapel Hill created a script to be used by bystanders, family members, and patients to alert them to the possibility of a stroke. If you suspect a stroke, ask the person to do three simple things:

1. Smile

2. Raise both arms and keep them up

3. Speak a simple sentence

The inability to carry out any one of these commands is the most common indication of a stroke. Attempts to smile result in obvious facial distortion because the facial muscles are weakened or paralyzed. A stroke patient may not be able to raise an arm because it also has been weakened. And he or she may have slurred or unintelligible speech.

You might be wondering where the researchers found enough subjects to evaluate this simple test. You can't stand in the street waiting for lots of people to have strokes. And you don't want to wish one on yourself. The researchers came up with an ingenious answer: Why not find some volunteers to test it on hospital patients who had recently had strokes? That's what they did. (I must say that these researchers had a little chutzpah. If I were in a hospital recovering from a stroke, I wouldn't welcome a bunch of strangers coming to my bedside and asking me to smile!)

The test itself had two goals: First, to see whether the average layman would be able to administer the test and interpret the results. Second, to determine whether the symptoms being evaluated really appear often enough in a stroke.

Here's what the researchers found: Of the 100 selected volunteers, 96 were able to administer the test properly. They detected arm weakness 95 percent of the time, facial weakness 71 percent of the time (I suppose that's because even normal faces can be asymmetrical), and slurred speech in 88 percent of patients. That's pretty good. I mean, we aren't exactly doing MRIs and CT scans of the brain!

THE BOTTOM LINE

Learn and apply these three simple steps when you or anyone else suddenly develops symptoms that raise the possibility of a stroke. If one or more are abnormal, get yourself or them to the hospital ASAP.

THYROID CANCER

· · · · · · · · · ·

Radiation Exposure and Potassium Iodide

SINCE SEPTEMBER 11, 2001, Americans have been conditioned to expect more terrorist attacks, especially a nuclear attack or radiation exposure from a faulty nearby nuclear facility.

Unfortunately, nothing will protect you if you're near ground zero and you receive a megadose of radiation. But if you do survive, you're at risk for thyroid cancer years later. That's what happened in Chernobyl when its power plant suffered a major leak. Most of the victims were kids who went on to develop thyroid cancer.

HERE'S WHAT'S NEW

The American Academy of Pediatrics is recommending that households, schools, and child care centers within 10 miles of a nuclear power plant keep potassium iodide pills on hand to protect children from accidental or intentional release of radiation. The Academy suggests stockpiling these pills even within a larger radius because of fallout that could be carried a greater distance downwind, such as that which occurred near Chernobyl.

Federal nuclear regulators have made potassium iodide available free of charge to states with nuclear plants, and these states have provided them to citizens deemed geographically vulnerable. Also, the U.S. Nuclear Regulatory Commission requires nuclear plants to stockpile potassium iodide to protect plant workers.

Potassium iodide blocks the thyroid gland's absorption of harmful radioactive iodine, which can cause cancer in the future. Children are more vulnerable to thyroid cancer from radioactive iodine fallout because their glands absorb and metabolize iodine more easily. When the children take potassium iodide pills, the iodine they contain is picked up by the thyroid, so that the gland is unable to handle any more iodine in radioactive form.

THE BOTTOM LINE

If you live within 15 miles of a nuclear plant, no one will think you're neurotic if you stock up on some potassium iodide, especially if you have children in your household. Play it safe, especially when it's so easy—and free. I'll let you in on a little secret: We have no kids at home anymore, but guess what? I keep a bottle of potassium iodide in our medicine chest.

These pills do not require a prescription, they have few if any adverse effects, and you can get them at a drugstore or on the Internet. If you don't open the bottle and keep it at room temperature, the pills maintain their potency indefinitely.

They work best when taken immediately after exposure. The dose is 130 milligrams for anyone weighing more than 154 pounds; those who weigh less should take half that amount. The recommended dose for children up to 1 month of age is 16 milligrams; for children 1 month to 3 years of age, it's 32 milligrams.

Taking thyroid supplements does not interfere with this pill. One dose of potassium iodide provides 24 hours of protection, by which time you should have hightailed it out of the area. Radioactive iodine remains in the environment for 8 days, so once you leave, you should stay away from home for at least that long. If you can't or won't leave, take the pills until there is no further risk of exposure to radioiodines.

THYROID DISEASE

· · · · · · · · · ·

The Great Imitator

THYROID DISEASE is sneaky business. It causes a surprising array of symptoms, all of which are easily attributable to some other cause. Take fatigue, the hallmark of low thyroid function. Who doesn't feel tired now and then? And many of us have trouble losing weight, or become constipated, or lose a little hair, or feel unusually cold, or develop dry skin. Aren't we all occasionally nervous or irritable? Conversely, many of us have trouble sleeping once in a while or experience a racing heartbeat—both symptoms of an overactive gland.

I don't want you to be a hypochondriac. However, you should know that if any of these common complaints persist, they may, in fact, reflect a treatable thyroid disorder. Over the years I have seen many patients who either were chronically tired and convinced that they were "born that way," or were very "high-strung" because, as they claimed, "that's my nature." Some of them were right, but many turned out to have either overfunction or underfunction of the thyroid—the gland that sets our "energystat." The appropriate treatment "miraculously" changed their lives.

The thyroid gland, located over the windpipe, makes two hormones that control heart rate, body temperature, vocal pitch, muscle strength, blood pressure, bowel function, mood, memory—even cholesterol level, and how often a woman menstruates.

Some 13 million Americans, eight times as many women as men, have a thyroid problem. At least half of them are unaware of it. By the time she reaches 60, one woman in five has an underactive thyroid gland, as do almost 10 percent of men at that age. In yet another twist, 8 percent of women develop a thyroid problem after they have had a baby.

The two major types of thyroid disorder are hypothyroidism and hyperthyroidism.

Hypothyroidism (an underactive gland) is by far the more common of the two. It explains the lack of "oomph" and energy in more than 11 million Americans, mostly women and the elderly. The symptoms usually start insidiously and worsen as time goes on.

It's important to recognize the telltale symptoms of hypothyroidism and intervene early. Even though you are sleeping, eating, and exercising correctly, you do have one or more of the following?

- Constant exhaustion

- Mild depression

- Weakness

- Constipation

- Dry, thick skin; decreased perspiration; dry scalp; coarse and thinning hair; and brittle nails

- Deepened vocal timbre
- Memory loss
- Difficulty losing weight
- Always feeling cold
- Thinning of the outer third of your eyebrows
- Increase in neck size
- Infertility, miscarriage, irregular periods with heavy bleeding, loss of sexual interest
- Climbing cholesterol level
- Decreased heart rate and blood pressure

By contrast, in hyperthyroidism (an overactive thyroid gland) there is too much thyroid hormone circulating in the bloodstream. Less common than an underactive gland, it affects 1 in every 100 Americans, including former president George H. W. Bush and his wife, Barbara. Almost 90 percent of these cases are women.

Suspect an overactive thyroid gland if you experience, and have no other explanation for, any combination of the following symptoms:

- Unusual and persistent restlessness
- Anxiety
- Mood swings
- Easy distractibility and inability to concentrate
- Increased tiredness, muscle weakness
- Skin that is warm, flushed, smooth, and moist
- Fine, silky, thin hair
- Increased perspiration
- Ravenous appetite but no weight gain

- Increased neck fullness below the Adam's apple
- Rapid heartbeat and palpitations
- Skipped heartbeats
- Shortness of breath after even slight exertion
- More frequent and usually soft bowel movements
- Irregular, scanty periods
- Bulging eyes; blurred and double vision
- A fine tremor in your hands and fingers
- Full, tender breasts (even in men)

Any combination of these symptoms suggests the possibility of hyperthyroidism. If your gland is hyperactive, you may develop a *thyroid storm or crisis at any time* (the pulse becomes very rapid, fever sets in, and you become agitated and possibly even delirious). This is a prime emergency.

Because thyroid disease is so prevalent and its symptoms often subtle, especially in the elderly, the American College of Physicians recommends that thyroid evaluation, done by a simple blood test, be part of the routine health examination of all men and women age 35 and older. I agree. One test in particular, the TSH level, is accurate and relatively inexpensive. It measures the amount of thyroid-stimulating hormone in the bloodstream. High TSH levels indicate hypothyroidism; low levels indicate hyperthyroidism.

HERE'S WHAT'S NEW

The best therapy for hypothyroidism is simply replacement of the missing hormone. This means taking a thyroid hormone pill every day. Thyroid replacement therapy almost always must be continued for life because hypothyroidism never "goes away."

The most frequently used therapy for hyperthyroidism is radioactive iodine (I-131), which you drink in a glass of water. It's odorless and tasteless, and it knocks out thyroid tissue, making it impossible for the gland to produce any of its hormones. It is 90 to 95 percent successful, but it takes several weeks to work. We used to worry that radioactive treatment, especially in young people, might lead to cancer of the thyroid later on. Long-term follow-up studies have not substantiated this fear.

If for any reason you prefer not to have the radioactive treatment, there is an acceptable alternative. Two antithyroid drugs stop production of thyroid hormone: propylthiouracil, usually taken three times a day; and methimazole, which is long-acting and you take it only once a day. They can occasionally cause a dangerous blood disorder, so you must have your blood checked every few months to be sure you're not among the unlucky one percent to whom this happens.

THE BOTTOM LINE

If you are either constantly tired or are "hopping" and irritable for no apparent reason, ask your doctor for the blood tests diagnose malfunction of the thyroid gland. Both overactive and underactive thyroid disorder can be easily treated and well tolerated.

URINARY TRACT INFECTION

· · · · · · · · ·

More Juice, Less Sex!

ABOUT 10 MILLION AMERICANS, most of them women, develop a urinary tract infection (UTI) every year. In many, the problem is recurrent. Men also suffer from UTIs, but much less frequently. There are several reasons for this difference. First, the urethra, the duct that carries the urine out of the body, is much shorter in women and its opening is close to the anus and vagina, both of which harbor the most common UTI-causing bacteria, *Escherichia coli* (*E. coli*). Women who use a diaphragm are more vulnerable to UTI. The risk of infection is even greater if their partner uses a condom with a spermicidal foam because these foams promote the growth of *E. coli*.

Tissues in the vagina, urethra, and bladder of menopausal women who lack estrogen become thinner making them vulnerable to irritation and infection. Diabetics are also more prone to UTIs because bacteria thrive in the glucose of the urine. So are children younger than age 2, whose soiled diapers are loaded with bacteria. Men who require catheterization because of prostate enlargement or for other reasons are also susceptible to UTIs.

Treating recurrent UTIs consists of removing the offending cause. Several antibiotics can then eradicate the infecting organisms. Drinking lots of fluids and avoiding alcohol also helps.

HERE'S WHAT'S NEW

Frankly, much of the following is not really new but does reinforce with impressive data what most people already suspected. For example, it's no secret that cranberry juice helps prevent recurrent UTIs. The news is that juice from several other berries also does so. If cranberry juice is not your cup of tea, you can also drink fresh juice from blueberries, raspberries, strawberries, lingonberries (I don't know anyone who's ever had lingonberry juice), cloudberries (ditto), and currants. Other fruit juices (apple, orange, grapefruit) are useful too, but are not nearly as effective as berry juices. Researchers at the University of Finland, found that whereas 1 to 3 glasses of these fruit juices a day reduced the incidence of UTIs in women by one-third, berry juices did so twice as often.

Berries work because they are rich in flavonols, compounds that make it hard for the germs in the urinary tract to attach themselves to the body's cells. As a result, they are washed away with the urine (the bacteria, that is, not the cells!).

It isn't only what you drink that's important. Certain foods such as sour cream, live-culture yogurt, and cheese are also helpful because they contain friendly bacteria that replace the harmful ones. Women who consume them at least three times a week have only one-fifth the incidence of UTIs as those who don't.

All of which brings us to the matter of sex. I wish I had better news for you. The more sex a woman has, the more vulnerable she is to UTIs. Specifically, sexual intercourse a minimum of three times a week triples the risk as compared to only once a week. This is the kind of prescription doctors don't like to give. Do with it what you will.

THE BOTTOM LINE

If you're prone to urinary tract infections, whether you're male or female, first eliminate any obvious cause. Diabetics should keep their blood glucose level under optimal control. Menopausal women may need vaginal estrogen suppositories to reduce dryness and irritation. Women should remember to wipe *away* from the vagina after a bowel movement. And learn to recognize the symptoms of a UTI so you can nip the infection in the bud with the appropriate antibiotics.

Get into the habit of drinking some kind of berry juice at least three times a week and eating yogurt two or three times a week, or both.

As far as sex is concerned avoid condoms coated with potentially irritating spermicides. And change from a diaphragm to another form of birth control. How often you have sex is entirely up to you. Personally, I wouldn't cut down. It isn't worth it!

UTERINE FIBROIDS

• • • • • • • • •

Avoid or Delay Surgery

UTERINE FIBROIDS are the most common benign tumors in women. They occur at any age in 25 percent of all females, usually before menopause, and are the leading reason for having a hysterectomy. Whether they cause symptoms (they do in about 40 percent of women older than age 35) depends on their number and their size. They can be as small as a pea or larger than a cantaloupe; they may be single or numerous.

Fibroids require treatment only if their symptoms are troublesome. If there are too many or they are too big, they may cause heavy menstrual bleeding, pelvic or lower back pain, frequent urination, a swollen or distended abdomen, painful or troublesome bowels movements, and difficulty becoming or staying pregnant.

Current treatment of fibroids includes:

Hormone therapy. Reducing estrogen levels in the body can decrease the size of the tumors.

Myomectomy. This surgical procedure removes only the fibroids, leaving the rest of the uterus intact. However, fibroids recur in 10 to 30 percent. It is possible for a woman to become pregnant after a myomectomy, but the procedure may affect fertility if it scars the uterus.

Hysterectomy (uterectomy). This is major surgery in which the uterus is removed. It results in infertility.

Fibroid embolization. This invasive but nonsurgical procedure is done using a local anesthetic. The patient can usually go home the same day. A tiny catheter is introduced into an artery reached through a small incision in the thigh. Microparticles injected through the catheter into the artery end up in the "feeder" blood vessels that supply the fibroid, blocking them, thus starving and shrinking the fibroid. Embolization has a 94 percent success rate in experienced hands; some premenopausal patients can remain fertile.

HERE'S WHAT'S NEW

There are some new observations about the embolization technique. Doctors at the University of Toronto found that among 555 women with fibroids who had this procedure and who wished to have babies someday, 14 went on to do so within 2 years. Although that figure isn't high, remember that the hysterectomy alternative means no babies at all.

There is news on the drug front as well. Mifepristone, better known as RU-486 (the so-called abortion pill), was approved by the FDA in 2000 for inducing abortion during the first 7 weeks of pregnancy. This drug has now been shown to shrink fibroids, too.

Doctors at the University of Rochester in New York found that as low a daily dose as 5 milligrams (600 milligrams are usually needed to cause abortion) can halve the size of fibroids within 6 months. At the same time this treatment improves such symptoms as bladder pressure, and pelvic and low back pain. Although higher doses of RU-486 can cause hot flashes, these are not as common with 5 milligrams a day.

THE BOTTOM LINE

Treatment with RU-486 may be a good alternative for women whose fibroids are enlarging and who do not require urgent surgical intervention—for example, if they are not bleeding heavily and becoming progressively more iron deficient. However, if more invasive therapy is required, I suggest you look into the embolization technique. If you're of childbearing age and want to have babies, your best choices to deal with the fibroids are myomectomy and embolization.

WRINKLES

. . . .

A New Wrinkle with Botox

BOTOX IS THE COSMETIC RAGE THESE DAYS, especially to remove the wrinkles that let people know how you really feel (I prefer to call them "scowl lines"). These injections work. I have seen their results on the faces of so many beautiful people who apparently never get angry.

HERE'S WHAT'S NEW

Dermatologists at the Weill Cornell Medical College have noticed that new wrinkles have appeared in some patients whose original wrinkles were successfully eliminated with Botox. Here's how and why it happens. According to the Cornell doctors, when a patient unwittingly scowls, muscles in the upper nose, middle eyebrow, and eyelid are called into play because the original ones in the forehead were paralyzed in order to remove the wrinkles. The involvement of these alternative muscles, if it occurs often enough, may create new wrinkles.

THE BOTTOM LINE

Botox injections must be repeated every few months. So in the weeks and months after your first treatment, examine your face carefully. If you see new wrinkles in previously unaffected areas, you have two choices: Don't bother getting more shots (they don't come cheap), or be prepared to have the newly involved areas "Botoxed," too.

EPILOGUE

. . . .

At this point, Bugs Bunny would have said, "That's all, folks." But I can't do that because there's no end to medical discoveries.

However, in the real world, we must consider publishing deadlines. Were it not for them, I could have gone on writing about all the wonderful and interesting findings that constitute *Healing Breakthroughs*.

Given these practical constraints, I have continued searching for breaking medical news up to the last moment before this book went to press. The latest information is contained in a series of bulletins in the section called "Hold the Presses!" that begins on page 379.

My goal is to keep you, my readers (all of whom I view as if you were my own patients), up to date on what's new and worthwhile in the field of human medicine. I expect to do so for as long as I can and for as long as you keep reading what I've written.

May every one of you find something in the foregoing pages that has made a difference to your health and well-being. Stay with it. It should be fun—and important.

HOLD THE PRESSES!

• • • • • • • • •

More red wine benefits. New research from Harvard suggests that red wine in moderation prolongs life by about 70 percent—at least in worms and fruit flies. This beneficial effect is presumed to be caused by resveratrol, a compound in the skin of the grape (and, incidentally, also in peanuts) that acts on other proteins to slow down or prevent cell death. The next step is to test these observations in rodents and eventually in humans.

Fish safety. Researchers at Stanford University, using newly available x-ray technology, have observed that the mercury in the muscle of fish is different and possibly less harmful than any of the other 26 known mercury compounds, each with its own toxicity profile. Scientists are cautiously optimistic that mercury in fish will be cleared of its present stigma, but they caution not to act yet on these initial observations.

Herpes help. The antiviral drug Valtrex (valacyclovir) substantially reduces the severity and duration of herpes infection as well as the incidence of its recurrence. The FDA has approved claims by the drug's manufacturer that it also decreases the chance of spreading the herpes infection to one's sexual partner by about 50 percent. Patients are still advised to avoid sexual contact during the characteristic flare-ups when sores reappear and to use condoms, although neither approach is foolproof.

Calcium to avenge Montezuma. Researchers in the Netherlands have found that subjects who were infected with a strain of *Escherichia coli*, the most common culprit in traveler's diarrhea, and received dietary calcium supplementation recovered 1 day sooner from their infection than did a control group. Their diarrhea was also less severe, and they lost less weight.

Mind over nausea. Researchers at the University of Rochester Medical Center evaluated acupressure wristbands for their effectiveness in controlling nausea in 700 cancer patients receiving chemotherapy. The wristbands had no effect on the nausea unless the patients expected them to be of help.

Botox for big prostates. Italian researchers injected Botox directly into the prostate glands of 15 men with symptoms of prostate enlargement. Men in a similar group were given placebo injections of saline. After 2 months, symptoms were reduced by 65 percent in 13 of the 15 Botox recipients. Only three of those who received the placebo said they felt better.

Another ACE inhibitor benefit. British researchers believe that people with uncomplicated coronary artery disease should take an angiotensin-converting enzyme (ACE) inhibitor in addition to a daily aspirin and a statin drug. They found that 12,000 patients given one of these medications had a 20 percent lower risk of cardiovascular death, heart attack, and cardiac arrest during the 4 years they were monitored. These doctors believed that adding the ACE inhibitor would prevent 100,000 heart attacks in their country with its population of 60 million.

Is your headache really migraine? Researchers at the Albert Einstein College of Medicine in New York have come up with three simple questions to help you identify whether your headache is a migraine. If you answer "yes" to two of the three questions, chances are you have migraine. The questions are: (1) Has a headache limited your activities for a day or more in the last 3 months? (2) Are you nauseated or sick to your stomach when you have a headache? (3) Does light bother you when you have a headache?

A UTI vaccine. Researchers at the University of Wisconsin Medical School have developed what they call "vaginal mucosal immunization" to prevent recurrent urinary tract infections in women. This vaccine takes the form of a vaginal suppository and may help prevent the emergence of antibiotic-resistant bacteria.

New uterine fibroid treatment. Doctors at five hospitals around the world including the Brigham and Women's Hospital in Boston have aimed ultrasound beams from outside the body to destroy fibroids. Patients require little pain medication, and they can go home the same day and return to work within a couple of days. This ultrasound technique looks promising, but it is still experimental. Doctors are not sure whether the fibroids will come back.

Good news for senior insomniacs. Researchers in the United States are enthusiastic about a new sleep medication called eszopiclone. (I am sure that its trade name, when announced, will be easier to remember and pronounce.) They found a 2-milligram dose to be effective, particularly in older people with a chronic sleep problem. It improved the quality and depth of slumber and increased the total sleep time. What's more, those who did awaken for any reason went back to sleep much more quickly.

A 3-minute hysterectomy. The FDA recently approved an amazing new alternative to hysterectomy. It's called microwave endometrial ablation and can be done as an outpatient procedure under light anesthesia. It involves using a handheld wand to emit high-frequency microwaves. It's fast (it takes 3 to 5 minutes), safe, and an effective alternative to surgery.

When to take Proscar. Recent research involving 19,000 men ages 55 and older at the University of Texas Health Sciences Center has shown that Proscar (finasteride), a drug used to treat symptoms of prostate enlargement, reduces the incidence of prostate cancer by nearly 25 percent. However, the drug did have a downside. Researchers observed that the cancers prevented by Proscar were small, probably insignificant ones, but that the number of life-threatening aggressive cancers increased.

Men, loosen your ties! British researchers reported in the *British Journal of Ophthalmology* that wearing a necktie too tight may increase the chance of developing glaucoma, an important cause of vision loss. In their experiments, these doctors found that tightening the tie raised eye pressure in 60 percent of men with glaucoma and 70 percent of normal males.

Medicare will pay for emphysema surgery. For people with advanced cases of emphysema, surgical removal of a portion of the diseased lung greatly improves quality of life. The average cost of such surgery and follow-up is $61,000. Medicare has announced that the benefit of such surgery is enough for them to pick up the tab, which is good news for those unable to afford the procedure on their own.

When to change hospitals. Suppose you suddenly develop chest pain due to a heart attack and you immediately go to the nearest emergency department. The treatment you receive will depend on what that particular hospital can deliver. There are two main choices. You can be given clot-busting drugs or have a balloon angioplasty, in which the fresh clot is removed opening the blocked artery. Recent research reported in the *New England Journal of Medicine* indicates that 14 percent of heart attack patients treated with clot-busting drugs either died, or had another heart attack or stroke within 30 days, compared with only 8 percent treated with angioplasty.

Unfortunately, only 15 percent of hospitals in this country have the catheterization laboratory needed to perform this procedure. The location of such a hospital nearest you is the kind of information you should have before an attack occurs. If you have the choice, that's where you should ask the ambulance crew to take you. One important finding in this study was that patients who were transferred for angioplasty *within 2 hours* had the same benefit as those who had it immediately.

Statins for your eyes, too. The combination of aspirin and a statin is an effective way to reduce your chances of developing a form of macular degeneration. Researchers at the University of California School of Medicine in San Francisco found that people who had taken a statin drug were 60 percent less likely to develop this eye problem (and were also 60 percent more likely to have been on a daily aspirin).

New treatment for interstitial cystitis? This chronic condition causes severe bladder pain in many women. A small study suggests that injecting a solution containing a bacterium called BCG into the bladder reduces symptoms in nearly 70 percent of patients.

Ban chromium picolinate? The Food Standards Agency, a group of independent scientists and doctors that advises the British government, has called for a ban on the supplement chromium picolinate on the grounds that it can cause cancer of the upper respiratory tract, lungs, and stomach. Chromium picolinate is widely used by athletes, body builders, and diabetics. However, according to a more recent study of people with type 2 diabetes, adding 1,000 micrograms of chromium picolinate to their diet increased their insulin sensitivity by almost 9 percent. No mention of the cancer issue was made in this new research.

Chelation for stented arteries. Coated stents placed in arteries that have been ballooned open reduces the incidence of their closure—but they're expensive. Copper chelation may provide a cheaper and even more effective solution.

No spuds during pregnancy? Researchers in Australia have found that harmful bacteria present in soil can infect potatoes and beets. When pregnant women who are genetically vulnerable to diabetes eat these foods, the bacteria they contain can destroy the insulin-producing cells of their newborn and cause diabetes.

Other effects of NSAIDs. It's well known that anti-inflammatory drugs such as Advil (ibuprofen) can cause stomach irritation and bleeding. Now, thanks to a new disposable little camera that you can swallow and that takes pictures as it travels down the intestinal tract, nonsteroidal anti-inflammatory drugs (NSAIDs) have been shown to affect the small intestine in the same way.

Calming "restless legs." Restless leg syndrome is a neurologic disorder that affects up to 10 percent of the population. It interferes with sleep and causes pain as well as an uncontrollable urge to move the legs. A drug called Requip (ropinirole) significantly improves symptoms and is well tolerated.

Carotid artery decision. Some plaques in the carotid arteries (in your neck) should be removed to prevent a stroke; others can safely be left alone. It's been the doctor's judgment call—until now. Early study results suggest that an MRI of the neck may be able to distinguish between those that can cause trouble and those that won't.

Nuts to you! Previous studies have shown that eating almonds improves your cholesterol and related blood levels. But the surprise is that despite their high energy content, almonds are not likely to cause weight gain. That's presumably because they promote increased excretion of fat in the stool.

Microwave those dentures. Just brushing and cleaning your dentures does not rid them of the bacteria and fungi that can cause sores and infections of the gums and mouth. You need to microwave them. If they have no metal components, put the dentures in a microwave container at least twice their height, with a vented lid. Fill the container with water and add a denture-cleaning tablet. Cover it with a towel, microwave for 2 minutes, then cool the dentures and rinse.

Warts away! Your kids will be happy with this one. The common warts so many of them have can now be removed by an over-the-counter aerosol spray that freezes them. Most warts then fall off within 10 days. If they don't, simply spray them again. No more visits to the dermatologist for liquid nitrogen.

Good bacteria for ulcerative colitis. If you're one of the 500,000 Americans with chronic ulcerative colitis, an inflammatory bowel disease (the other is Crohn's disease), a novel treatment has been shown to be effective. VSL#3 is a combination of 450 billion harmless bacteria (such as lactobacillus), which, taken by mouth, helps balance the intestinal bacterial population that may be infecting and inflaming your gut. In a recent trial, 86 percent of 30 patients with this problem responded to this treatment.

Keep your nitroglycerin. Doctors have always told their patients that nitroglycerin tablets (the little white pills that are used to treat angina and dissolve under the tongue) should be discarded 6 months after the bottle has been opened. That's no longer necessary. The pills have now been reformulated so you can keep them until the expiration date on the bottle. And, of course, you may prefer to take your nitroglycerin in the form of a spray under the tongue.

Alpha-lipoic acid and diabetes. *Polyneuropathy*—numbness, pain, tingling of the extremities—is a common and difficult-to-treat complication of long-standing diabetes. According to new research, a daily dose of 600 milligrams of the antioxidant alpha-lipoic acid improved these symptoms after 3 weeks in more than half the patients treated.

Drink to prevent diabetes. Diabetes can be prevented in men and women by drinking four or more cups of coffee a day, mainly because of the caffeine. However other ingredients in the brew may play a part as well, since decaffeinated coffee also works (but to a lesser extent). Moderate intake of beer and wine also cuts the risk of diabetes, but only in women. However, heavy drinkers have a greater incidence of the disease.

Cut the cost of Lipitor in half! The cost of drugs in the United States is prohibitive and often beyond the financial ability of many patients, especially those who are retired and on a fixed income. Changes in Medicare may not become effective for at least 2 years. Recent research indicates that at least for Lipitor (atorvastatin), one of the most commonly used drugs to lower cholesterol levels, taking the pill every other day instead of daily has the same effect on blood levels. Check with your doctor to see whether this applies to other members of the statin family of medications.

New drug adds height. In the past 16 years, growth hormone has been administered to 200,000 children worldwide who were extremely short because they had growth-stunting disease or their bodies were not producing enough growth hormone. The FDA has agonized for years whether this hormone should be given to more of these short children. Now, it has finally approved the administration of growth hormone somatropin (Humatrope, made by the Eli Lilly Company) when growth patterns suggest that a boy will not be taller than 5 feet 3 inches and a girl no more than 4 feet 11 inches. In such cases you can expect an additional 1.5 to 2.8 inches. When considering its use for your children, you should know that Humatrope must be injected six times a week for several years and costs between $10,000 and $25,000 a year. What's more, it is only available at selected drug stores, and can be prescribed only by designated specialists.

INDEX

· · · · · · · · · ·

Underscored page references indicate boxed text.